The Official YMCA Fitness Program

D1224725

The Official YMCA Fitness Program

Compiled and edited by the National Board of YMCAs
under the direction of William B. Zuti, Ph.D.,
National Director of Health Enhancement

RAWSON ASSOCIATES
NEW YORK

Any fitness program involving exercise and diet should be
undertaken only with the approval and under the supervision of
your physician.

Library of Congress Cataloging in Publication Data

National Board of the Young Men's Christian Associations.
The official YMCA fitness program.

Includes index.
1. Physical fitness. 2. Exercise. I. Zuti, William B.
II. Title. III. Title: Official Y.M.C.A. fitness program.
GV481.N27 1984   613.7   83-42630
ISBN 0-89256-253-6
ISBN 0-89256-254-4 (pbk.)

Packaged by Sandra Choron, March Tenth, Inc.
Composition by Folio Graphics Co., Inc.
Printed and bound by Fairfield Graphics, Fairfield, Pennsylvania
Designed by Stanley S. Drate
First Edition

CONTENTS

SECTION A
Fitness

SECTION **B**

Food

"Wellness, feeling good, is an active process of becoming aware of what is possible not only in the physical but in all dimensions of life."

Dr. William Hettler, Director of
University Health Services,
University of Wisconsin at
Stevens Point, and a lifelong
YMCA volunteer

Rather than indulge in false modesty, we will say simply that the YMCA feels eminently qualified to give advice and instruction on attaining sound physical health through exercise, sports, and proper nutrition. What's more, the Y considers itself no less suited to counsel on the positive effect of physical fitness on emotional health. After all, these areas have been the YMCA's very reason for existence over all its long history.

The YMCA began in London, England, in 1844 as a response to the Industrial Revolution, which was then in its dynamic formative years. Western man was becoming rapidly urbanized by the shift to factory and office employment. Work required less and less physical exertion and was much more enervating than the pastoral rhythms he had followed in the not-too-distant past. This "tension of modern times" was compounded and magnified by his having to live in crowded cities, where there were practically no outlets for the physical exercise he was missing.

The very first founders of the YMCA initially concerned themselves only with the "spiritual and mental condition of commercial young men" and organized regular meetings for discussions of "mental culture" and general good fellowship. But soon after—particularly in the United States—the concept of the "whole man" began to take root in the YMCA movement, whereby mental powers and spiritual stability were seen as being one with physical health.

The YMCA's first step in developing its physical education/fitness program was to install a bowling alley in its Brooklyn, New York, building. The rationale for this simple beginning was rather quaintly stated: "Men whose principal occupation is brainwork need muscular amusement." Within a few years YMCAs began building gymnasiums and pools. By the turn of the century YMCAs were well established as the leading physical education organization in the United States.

Today, of course, the YMCA is a vast and sophisticated organization with extensive facilities throughout the United States and in many other countries around the world. To think YMCA is to think gymnasium, basketball, racquetball, swimming pools, exercise rooms, summer camp, and, in general, a congenial surrounding that enhances the pursuit of a sound body and frame of mind. We are proud of this synergistic connection.

Such growth has not been accidental, and certainly not for lack of competition. The YMCA also takes pride in having inspired the birth of other major organizations devoted to the same end, such as the YWCA (Young Women's Christian Association), the CYO (Catholic Youth Organization), the YMWHA (Young Men's and Women's Hebrew Association), and the Jewish Community Centers. The YMCA has thrived as the result of a concentrated and continuing effort to achieve its basic aims through tried and true methods, but at the same time it has always been willing and enthusiastic to try new ways to "get old age dancing itself young," as someone once put it with charming informality.

In short, the YMCA has never stood pat. It is always open to fresh ideas and information in the pursuit of bodily health and its intimate connection with mental and spiritual activity and development. Accordingly, this book incorporates all that the YMCA has found to be successful over the years, plus the most recent discoveries in the areas of physical fitness, nutrition, and mental well-being.

ACKNOWLEDGMENTS

This book would not be possible without the hard work and dedication of literally thousands of YMCA staff and volunteer leaders. The final copy was edited by Al Barkow, who spent countless hours polishing the manuscript. The illustrations were carefully drawn by Laura D'Argo.

INTRODUCTION

More and more Americans are making the exciting discovery that exercise makes them feel good and that they like the feeling of feeling good. In its two thousand branches the YMCA alone has over 12 million members and participants who are pursuing good health.

But is it exercise alone that produces this exhilaration? Not quite. At the core, certainly, are the various exercises and athletic activities that improve the cardiovascular system, stretch muscles, increase strength and endurance, and create a leaner physical profile. But exercise also stimulates the development of what might be called an integral support system, one that both enlarges and enriches the entire fitness process. The support system includes the food we eat and an attitude that helps us to withstand emotional stress and form more satisfying relationships with people.

That may seem like a lot to expect from bent-knee sit-ups, head and hip rotations, jogging, and swimming, but studies have proven many times over that the way we act and the way we feel about ourselves and others are profoundly influenced by our physical condition. In the end, the three elements—or roads—of fitness, food, and attitude converge to form a single highway. This idea of integration is the essential theme of the YMCA and thus of this book, making it unique among the many books on health that are available today.

The Motivation to Feel Good

Just about everyone will accept at face value that exercise and good nutrition are good for them. Yet this is not always enough to induce people to start a regulated physical fitness program. What prompts some people to do so and keeps others from it? One answer involves what sociologists call peer pressure. We may decide to improve our physical condition because others in our group place a high value on it and are doing so themselves; or we may decide *not* to because our compatriots—family and/or friends—are not interested in fitness and might even resent those who are.

The latter situation is of great concern to fitness leaders of the YMCA. Many people do make a personal decision to break with their peers. The challenge for them is to stay on course by finding a new support group and coping with the impact or threat their life-style changes may impose on the people around them.

Coping strategy is a subject we will discuss at length in the section of this book on attitude. For now we will say only that the problem has been resolved many more times than not, to everyone's satisfaction and growth as human beings. Every YMCA is full of men and women of all ages who are struggling with this issue and who are winning together.

Regardless of how the decision to get physically fit affects our personal relationships, we believe that making the decision to be healthy must be based in very large part on well-established facts and figures. More people know how the human body works (and doesn't work) than at any time in man's history. It would be foolish to ignore the knowledge that the sciences have provided.

What have we learned about ourselves that we can apply to achieving physical well-being? Most important, we know that every second death in the United States is cardiovascular in origin and that coronary heart disease—the classic "heart attack"—accounts for most of that statistic. The remainder is attributed to ailments related to blood circulation: stroke, atherosclerosis, and hypertension. This plight has arisen not only in the group traditionally disposed to heart trouble—men in middle age and beyond—but also among women, young people, and even children.

In the past the heart attack was blamed primarily on sudden exertion and heavy emotional stress, and such shocks and strains can surely bring it on. At the YMCA, however, we have come to realize that the groundwork for heart attack is laid by general physical deterioration over an extended period of time. Today's heart attack began perhaps ten years ago with an unspoken decision *not* to take care of your physical welfare. Of course, some physical deterioration is linked to aging and cannot be avoided. On average, for example, a sixty-year-old person has about 70 percent of the maximum oxygen uptake of a twenty-five-year-old. (Oxygen uptake is the amount of oxygen that can be transported to the body tissues from the lungs; it is one of the most highly regarded measures of a person's capacity for work.) But the inevitable ebbing of the life force can be slowed with proper diet and exercise.

World-renowned authority on physical medicines, Professor Per-Olof Astrand has worked with the YMCA for the past fifteen years and has been the keynote speaker at three major YMCA national health and fitness conferences in the United States. He points out:

"If two fifty-year-olds are identical in [physical] endowment but one is trained (i.e., systematically exercised) and the other is untrained, the trained person will have an oxygen uptake ability—and maximum motor power—on the same level as the untrained person had at around the age of thirty-five to forty. In other words, *moderate training* can lead to a ten-to-fifteen-year biological rejuvenation."

Can there be a more compelling motive for getting into a physical fitness program?

Professor Astrand's "moderate training" revolves around calisthenics, especially aerobic exercises such as brisk walking, swimming, jogging, cycling, skipping rope, and cross-country skiing. The YMCA has learned from experience that aerobic exercises are far more effective than anaerobic exercises for conditioning the cardiovascular system and contributing to weight control. In fact, we do not recommend anaerobics such as heavy weight lifting by itself for average men and women beyond their college years who are not competitive athletes either on professional or highly skilled amateur levels.

What Is "Physically Fit?"

We want to make it very clear from the outset that every individual has his/her own physical capabilities and limitations. We realize as well that bodies come in all sizes and shapes.

There are, however, general averages for cardiovascular efficiency, flexibility, and the amount of body fat a person should have. We present detailed tables on this information. But we want to stress the idea that these averages are only general guides and that each of you must set goals for personal well-being that take into account your particular physical history.

One important aspect of your history is heredity. Each of us must be very much aware of the physical characteristics of our relatives. Genetics plays no small role in how you are made, how your body can or will function, what you eat and how much of it, and even how you may think about yourself.

Because you are unique unto yourself, you should not get into a competition with others or with the charts in order to reach what amounts to idealized fitness goals. You must compete only against yourself and achieve an *individual fitness level.*

At the same time, your level of fitness is not entirely arbitrary. We will tell you why you must take a thorough physical examination from your doctor and a fitness evaluation from a trained fitness counselor before embarking on an exercise program. It is important to know how fit you are at the moment and how fit you can expect to become. Professionals in the field of health are best qualified and equipped to tell you. However, the YMCA has found that the participants must take responsibility for themselves once they begin an exercise program. You will not stay in shape by being dependent on "pros." Fitness can be measured by numbers, and we show you how to count them. We teach you to keep your fitness score—how to measure your pulse rate, keep track of your strength and endurance level, your flexibility, and how much fat you are carrying.

Working Out Need Not Be Work

Many people believe exercise is a chore, that all the bending and stretching may be good for them but is too boring and becomes merely a task. What's more, some people think that exercises will do you good only if they are done under the supervision of a browbeating expert with the style of an army drill sergeant. Thus the decision to get into exercise gets "postponed" indefinitely.

We acknowledge that calisthenics can become monotonous. But YMCAs have added music to most fitness classes and recruited leaders with far more exciting personalities than the old "drill sergeant." We also suggest that the intrapersonal competition we spoke of should be used in doing calisthenics. By competing against yourself to achieve daily, weekly, annual, and lifetime fitness goals the calisthenics become a game.

But we would also like to appeal to a somewhat higher sense of yourself. Think of the chin-ups, push-ups, and other exercises as trees of a grand forest—good health—and they become vital reasons for being or doing.

There are alternatives to calisthenics—exercise machines, to name but one. The YMCA does not think the machines are the be-all-end-all of exercise, but they are a popular aid for personalized exercise. They allow you to exercise all the vital body parts, and while much of this can be accomplished with regular calisthenics, there is a certain pleasure in performing on the machines. They have a technological appeal that suits our times.

Since very few people can afford to own these machines, they are most often used in an organizational setting such as a YMCA. Other people are going through the line at the same time, so there is a degree of sociability that accrues. In any case, we shall illustrate and describe the exercise machines and advise you on how and how much to use them.

The most satisfying alternative to calisthenics is participation in sports and games. We divide this into four categories: aquatics, which include such on-the-water activities as canoeing and rowing and such in-the-water ones as swimming; racket games, such as tennis, squash, and racquetball; pedal sports, such as jogging, running, hiking, and climbing; and ball games, such as volleyball, basketball, and handball. The YMCA operates more swimming pools than any other organization in the country. Youth and adult sports leagues were originated by the YMCA—the inventor of both basketball and volleyball.

Any of the above are very enjoyable both emotionally and intellectually, and they will also exercise your body. But many of the sports and games fall short of the full range of exercises. For instance, jogging is an excellent aerobic exercise, but it does not work out the muscles of the arms, back, or abdomen. For this reason we believe everyone should combine certain calisthenics with his/her sports or games to get a full-rounded workout. We suggest what combinations will fulfill this.

Go It Alone, If You Wish

It is not absolutely necessary to take exercise in a group situation or outside your own home. This applies mainly to calisthenics, which obviously can be done in private. However, everyone should get some advice from a fitness expert at least when starting a program, as well as a complete physical examination from a doctor. Naturally, if you find it difficult to get or remain motivated to exercise in existential solitude, and that is not uncommon, you can always join a group. We will illustrate how calisthenics taken in a group setting can be an enjoyable social event, a venue for expanding your range of friendships by sharing the same ambition—good health.

Food and You

There is another misconception about the pursuit of well-being that has to do with nutrition. Many people think that eating properly means giving up all the foods they enjoy and taking up exotic special diets composed of things never before thought to be fit for human consumption. It is understandable how this notion might develop, what with the welter of diet books that are trumpeted as *the* solution to getting and staying thin.

In fact, though, a great many of these high-flown, overblown fad diets will end up putting weight on your frame, and some can be downright dangerous to your health. We will explain this and present the YMCA line of thinking on nutrition: eat pretty much what you like from all four food groups, just a little *less* of it, and *always combine eating with exercise.* We also present tables on how many calories certain foods have and how many minutes of certain exercises will burn them off.

This is not to say we think it is okay to eat foods loaded with refined sugar, sodium, fat, and cholesterol. In all, people would be better off without these elements in their diet—or at least with a lot less. But they need not be avoided entirely. We believe eating is not only to stoke a furnace. It should also give pleasure and satisfaction to the taste buds. To help you formulate a nutritious diet, we will provide comprehensive tables detailing the nutritional values of our basic foodstuffs, the vitamins and minerals they contain, why additives are put into them, and whether these additives are safe or unsafe to eat.

We will also discuss the hereditary and sociocultural influences on our eating habits. For example, overweight is one of the major causes of heart trouble, and almost half the American population is overweight. Why? Mainly because people eat too much fat-producing food and do not exercise enough to burn it off. And why is that?

Before the twentieth century, overweight was not much of a problem for most people. People did not store up great quantities of fat because the natural course of their lives did not allow it. Most work for men—in the fields and other occupations—and for women in the home was strenuous enough to keep everyone reasonably lean and trim. But modern technology has caused us to substitute brain for brawn, so that over 50 percent of today's work force in the United States has sedentary jobs. More and more of us are doing a lot of sitting while earning our keep. Even the arduous occupations that still exist, such as forestry, farming, construction, and factory work, require less and less real physical labor due to the advent of power tools, robots, and computers.

Inevitably, there has been a carryover from the workplace to our private lives and leisuretime. Just as we use highly sophisticated, automated equipment on the job, so we drive our cars around the corner to do a simple errand, ride motorized cars on the golf course, open cans of food by electricity, and may soon be ordering those cans from the market by home computer to be delivered to our doorstep.

Not only has this "easy life" led to a generally poor physical condition, it has brought on emotional unease. We seem to be more easily stressed now, and many people eat impulsively in an attempt to relax emotionally. Because the eating is a compensation for feeling bad, the diet is indulgent. Thus Americans eat enormous amounts of fat- and sugar-filled foods, drink rivers of highly sweetened soft drinks, and fill up on processed foods heavy in calories and dubious chemical adulterants. As a result, in such an immensely productive country as the United States, which is capable of supplying the best food in the world in huge quantities, a large part of the population suffers from malnutrition—not for the lack of something to eat, but for the lack of enough nutrition in the food that is eaten.

To understand the genesis of our eating habits, as well as the ingredients of our food, is to take a giant first step toward making changes for the better.

The Stress Factor

We have mentioned stress, and how many people eat—usually poorly—to relieve it. Another way people try to ease chronic butterflies in the stomach, tension headaches, and backache due to emotional upset is through seemingly constant change. Americans change their residence an average of every two years, and jobs about as often. Sometimes there is no choice, but in many cases the moves seem to be self-imposed nervous responses to deep-seated feelings of dissatisfaction. On the day-to-day level there is another symbol of this constant search. Many people now have remote-control push-button consoles with which they can punch up thirty or more television/cable channels in a minute, creating a mind-boggling montage of visual and audio images. Such a rate of change only incites more stress.

We point out such examples to support our view that one of the best ways to manage stress is through physical exercise. We examine stress in its most common forms and indicate how exercise and improved nutrition can reduce it significantly, if not altogether. We will describe, for instance, the biological process by which exercise causes a steady, balanced flow of adrenalin that thereby stems the rise of emotional tension.

The Partnering Concept

We have mentioned that one result of a person starting a serious effort at improving his/her physical fitness can be difficult interpersonal relationships. One means of avoiding such a problem can be through family or friends' involvement in your program, even if the participation does not include exercising. We will show how and why such "partner-ing" has worked successfully for many.

We also point out the growth in corporate health programs that are being delivered in the workplace, or through it, which have a valuable "partnering" effect. The YMCA is deeply involved in this area.

Most people probably know a good bit about what we have said here about exercise and nutrition and the problems of stress. If they don't know in detail, surely they do in an intuitive way. And many have begun doing something corrective. There has been a substantial move toward exercise and better nutrition. It appears the tide is beginning to turn in favor of fitness.

We understand that no one is going to make a wholesale retraction of his modern life-style. We don't expect people to return to using the horse-drawn, hand-held plow, to bring themselves water by the bucket from a deep well, to eat only fresh-picked fruits and vegetables and fresh-killed meat. On the other hand, the human body has not changed very much in the last few thousand years. It still functions as it always has, so we have only to amend our care and feeding of it by going back to basics.

The "basics" is physical exercise, which is not at all a new idea either. The citizens of ancient Greece were perhaps the first people to examine thoroughly the human body and reveal some of its mysteries. The Greeks of the Golden Age understood the value of physical exercise and practiced it assiduously, performing many of the calisthenics that are included in this book. What is more, in their art the ancient Greeks glorified the human form as it had never been done before. They produced multidimensional sculptures of men and women, those elegant figures of gods and goddesses that to this day represent to us the anatomical ideal.

Also from this enlightened civilization came the striking body of intellectual thought that is the foundation of our thinking today in science, art, philosophy. Thus the essential thrust of this book is but a reaffirmation of the classic unity of mind and body in the full exercise of each.

Luther H. Gulick, M.D., was a member of the faculty at the YMCA College in Springfield, Massachusetts, in 1887 when he focused the attention of the YMCA on the integration of body, mind, and spirit. He developed the YMCA triangle as the symbol of the need to work with the whole person. The YMCA has been in the business of helping people develop healthy life-styles for over one hundred years.

SECTION A

Fitness

1

What Is Physical Fitness?

Contrary to what Hollywood casting directors have led us to believe over the years, the tall and lean cowboy sitting high in the saddle is not necessarily stronger and quicker—not necessarily as physically fit—as the short, stocky fellow pushing a plow over the "back forty." And if he isn't, it may well be because he doesn't push a plow for a living. But that is another matter, which we deal with elsewhere in this book. The point here is that physical fitness cannot be defined by surface appearances, especially those that are the result of heredity.

Each of us has been given at birth a set of essential genetic characteristics that cannot be altered. We will be tall or short or somewhere in between because our ancestors were tall or short or somewhere in between. While you may be perfectly fit, in excellent health, you won't be able to run as fast as someone else in the same good condition simply because you have shorter legs or the width of your pelvis won't allow you greater speed. Some people have a naturally higher maximum oxygen uptake than others, and thus have more success in endurance competitions than those not similarly endowed; it might be the person with the shorter legs.

No exercise or special diet is going to change your genetic facts of life. It is important that you understand and accept this as you embark on a program to improve your physical health. It plays a definite role in your setting realistic goals for yourself.

However, while we may not be able to alter received physical traits permanently, we can surely modify them as we see fit. A striking example of this can be taken from big-time sports. When the great golfer Jack Nicklaus first came onto the professional tournament golf stage, he was a rather heavy young man. His physique, wide from top to bottom, resembled that of his father, who weighed well over 200 pounds. It was easy to see that the son would, or could, become the "spittin' image" of his dad in a few years.

In his very first year as a professional, Nicklaus won golf's most prestigious title, the U.S. Open, defeating Arnold Palmer in a play-off in such fashion that made it clear he would be a major force in his game for some time. Yet Nicklaus was not a popular winner; quite the opposite. The golfing public's generally negative reaction to Nicklaus' victory was in good part because he defeated a much adored hero figure. Palmer's defeat at the hands of a fellow eleven years his junior was a big disappointment, especially since Nicklaus won in such a convincing way and carried himself with great self-confidence—some would say arrogance. Although Nicklaus had every right to feel sure of himself, he received an unusually resentful response from the golfing gallery, which focused its feelings on Nicklaus' physical appearance. This contrasted sharply, by the way, with Palmer's thin-waisted, muscular, "athletic" figure. Nicklaus was called Fat Jack.

This was a trying time for Nicklaus, although it didn't seem to faze his competitive performance. Nonetheless, after a couple of seasons he decided to lose weight. During a long break from the tournament circuit he went on a program of careful eating and controlled exercises. Afterward, the "new" Jack Nicklaus appeared as an attractively slimmed down—albeit still solidly built—version of the same great golfer. Almost immediately the golfing public's reaction to Nicklaus changed for the better, and he subsequently became a very popular and totally accepted champion.

Would Nicklaus be lionized as he has, and would he have won as many championships, if he had remained "Fat Jack?" That is hard to say for sure, but Nicklaus unquestionably understood the dangers of overweight, not to say the taste of a public that likes its champion athletes to "look the part." It is not too much of a stretch of the imagination to assume that because he did not let himself grow in size to be as big as his father, who died of cancer at age fifty-six, Jack Nicklaus helped himself become "the greatest golfer in the history of the game." Nicklaus modified his genetic heritage and perhaps simultaneously mastered his game and gained the personal popularity everyone desires.

Sometimes such modifications of heritage as Jack Nicklaus imposed on himself have to be commanded by others. Case in point: military training. Those who have been in the service know, through personal experience or by observing their fellow servicemen, that during the basic training period trainees who are overweight at the beginning are trimmed down by the end of the course, and those who are underweight gain pounds. In each case an ideal weight-to-physique ratio is attained. This occurs because everyone eats meals designed by professional dieticians that provide all the required nutrition in the correct amounts (although the taste may not be applauded by the recruits), and everyone gets plenty of exercise—all that marching, calisthenics, field maneuvers. No doubt the regular hours have something to do with it, too.

A military basic training course runs only about six weeks and is more intensified than the schedule you are going to follow to reach your personal level of fitness. But the essential process is the same: a combination of proper diet and sufficient exercise.

How do you know what your "personal level of fitness" is? Hereditary factors aside, there are standards that have been set. For all the variety in physical structure among mankind, our physiological system is *generally* very much one; we have yet to discover any one of us without a rib cage or a heart that pumps blood. Thus, we provide tables showing the *average* heart rate, maximum oxygen uptake, and percentage of fat a person should have in relation to his or her total weight. We present many other tables giving averages we can use as guides. You do not have to match up exactly with any of them.

But before you can even begin to read these tables and work toward the averages, you must find out what kind of physical condition you are in at the moment and what your maximum fitness potential is. Out of this can be prescribed the sort of exercises you can and cannot do. How strong is your heart? What is your blood pressure? How much fat are you presently carrying on your frame? It is very important to have this information. Your safety, as well as your health, depends on it. To find out these and other things about your health and physical condition, you must have a thorough medical checkup and evaluation from a physician. You should also have a physical fitness evaluation administered by a trained fitness counselor. The latter is a part of any fitness program conducted at a YMCA. Even if you decide to "go it alone" in raising your fitness level, it is highly recommended you get some direction from a professional in the field.

Of the two preliminary checkups, *the physician's examination must come first.* In the following paragraphs we point out what the medical and fitness evaluations are meant to find and how this information is obtained.

Medical Evaluation

The medical evaluation involves a check of your family and personal health history, including current habits such as smoking, alcohol intake, diet, habitual physical activity, and working environment.

Special emphasis is put on finding a history of chest discomfort or pain, shortness of breath, and other signs related to cardiovascular or pulmonary (chest) disease. A standard electrocardiogram (ECG) test, taken when you are in a resting state, will probably detect problems in these areas. But if you are over thirty-five or have a family history of cardiovascular problems, the YMCA prefers you take a Stress ECG test. A Stress ECG test is taken while you are pumping a stationary bicycle or walking on a treadmill. It is a much surer way of discovering hidden heart trouble. Between 8 and 14 percent of the normal population who are without common symptoms of heart disease will show abnormalities when the heart is put under stress.

Also to be noted in a medical exam are orthopedic problems such as bone and joint abnormalities and a history of any bone breakage, for any of these can limit and/or determine the type of exercise to be taken.

If you expect to control your diet in conjunction with the exercise program, as most people tend to do, have the doctor determine your cholesterol count. Find out how much cholesterol you have in your system.

The physician should know what kind of exercise program you intend to participate in, and in his report make any recommendations in that regard. The doctor's report should be given to your fitness counselor.

Physical Fitness Evaluation

The YMCA has administered over a million physical fitness evaluations in the past decade. From this experience we can speak with authority about this important prerequisite to a new life-style. There are four areas by which physical fitness is evaluated. They are: Flexibility, Muscular Strength and Endurance, Cardiorespiratory Endurance and Efficiency, and Body Composition. Some of the tests in these areas are often administered by a doctor, such as blood pressure and heartbeat rate, but they can also be performed by a trained fitness counselor.

All the fitness test "scores" should be kept on a special sheet so regular monitoring of progress is possible.

The tests are in the following order:

Standing Height
Weight
Resting Heart Rate
Resting Blood Pressure
Body Composition (degree of fatness)
Cardiovascular Evaluation
Flexibility Measurement
Muscular Strength and Endurance

The following is a summary of each test so you know what is being looked for and why. There should be no mysteries in any of this, no secrets for experts only.

STANDING HEIGHT

This is not really a measure of physical fitness and can be eliminated. However, it is very easy to administer and helps describe the individual, so why not.

WEIGHT

This should be recorded while wearing a gym outfit, but no shoes. There will be considerably more on this subject under the Body Composition heading.

RESTING HEART RATE

This should be recorded while sitting, and several minutes after any sort of exercise has been completed.

RESTING BLOOD PRESSURE

This should also be recorded while sitting, and when you are well rested.

BODY COMPOSITION

This pertains to the amount of fat you have in your body. Everyone must have some fat as a nutritional reserve. It helps fight against periods of cold weather, provides energy during periods of vigorous physical activity, and staves off hunger because fat does not break down as quickly as protein and carbohydrates. Fat is also necessary for the metabolic and endocrine systems to function properly.

The real question is, how much fat should we have in our system? The generally accepted normal percentage of fat for males is 14 to 16 percent of total body weight. For females, who by nature have more fatty tissue than men, the normal percentage is between 23 and 26 percent of body weight.

You will notice we refer to the ratio of body fat to total body weight. The conventional, old-fashioned means for determining if someone was overweight was to match weight to height. But that is no longer satisfactory. It does not give a true picture. One person six feet tall and weighing 200 pounds may be overweight, whereas another person the same height and weight may be normal. The overweight person has more—too much—fat.

Height and weight charts do not reflect the percentage of fat in a person. Nor do they distinguish between bone and muscle. A demonstration of what we mean occurred at a large metropolitan police department, which had height and weight limitations for its officers. The maximum allowable weight for a six-footer was 210 pounds; anyone above this was considered overweight and subject to suspension. Indeed, two officers were suspended for being six feet tall and over 210 pounds. But both were well-conditioned bodybuilders and had only 19 percent fat in their bodies. Only after considerable explanation of the difference the amount of fat makes in a person's physical health, and that this is the true measure of a person's condition, were the officers reinstated.

At the YMCA we estimate total body fat by skinfold measurements. You can do this yourself either with a calipers designed for the purpose or simply with your fingers.

When we gain fat, much of it settles in certain parts of the body. This subcutaneous fat (fat below the skin surface) can be pinched up by the thumb and forefinger. As you get fatter, the skinfolds you pinch up get larger.

Skinfold calipers have a constant-tension spring so that regardless of how wide the jaws are spread, the tension between them is constant. To use the calipers, pinch up a skinfold and grasp it between the caliper jaws. A reading will register on the attached meter. A fitness counselor is adept at using the calipers. You may need some practice with them before you get sound readings, but it isn't that hard to get the hang of it.

If you don't want to spend money for a calipers, you can pinch up a skinfold with one hand, say in the area just above your waist, and measure it with the fingers of your other hand. Hold those fingers together and lay them across the top of the skinfold. If it takes only one finger to cover the fold, you are pretty trim. If it takes three fingers, you probably have too much fat. This of course is not the most scientific way to find out your body composition, but it gives you a general idea.

There are seven skinfold sites where fat usually accumulates. At least three of them for women and four for men should be measured to get a reliable estimate of overall body fat. The sites are illustrated on these pages, and we have also included a Fat and Target Weight Table for reference. However, a basic interpretation is quite simple. For example, if an individual has an abdominal skinfold of 28 mm at the start of a fitness program and reduces this to 18 mm in twenty weeks, he has a reduction of 10 mm of fat overall.

As already noted, for general good health an average male should have around 14 to 16 percent of fat, and the average female between 23 and 26 percent. From the standpoint of aesthetics or athletic training, however, men and women can be under those norms. Many male marathon runners, for instance, are from 10 to 12 percent fat. On the other hand, male weight lifters and football players tend to be 19 to 20 percent fat.

In any event, the average male with over 25 percent fat and the average female with over 35 percent are considered obese. Obesity, of course, is very much a potential health hazard.

Low fat content, however, does not necessarily mean low total weight. Muscle is heavier than fat, and if most of your total weight is in muscle, you are healthy. Low fat does mean fewer inches around the waist, though, because fat takes up more space than muscle.

By the way, fat cannot be changed to muscle, as a lot of people untrained in physical fitness seem to think. This idea apparently comes from the observation that when people lose body fat, they simultaneously become more muscular while total body weight remains the same. But loss of weight and increase of muscle tissue are separate events that occur at the same time. It follows, of course, that muscle does not turn to fat; it just gets soft and flabby.

THE SKINFOLD TEST FOR BODY COMPOSITION (FATNESS)

The seven skinfold sites for testing are shown below. In the procedure the skinfold should be lifted two or three times before being measured to make sure you have only fat and no muscle. Hold the skinfold firmly with the thumb and forefinger and place the caliper jaws below them. When the needle on the meter stops moving, you have your reading. Record the reading for each site.

We have also included a Body Composition Rating Scale for each of the skinfold sites and an overall Weight to Body Fat Table for men and women.

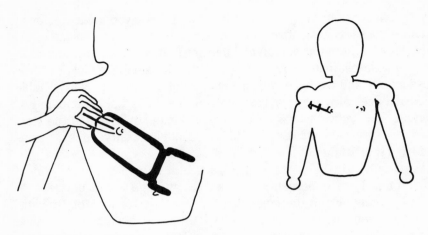

Skinfold Site 1—Chest (Pectoral)
A diagonal fold on the pectoral line midway between the axillary fold and the nipple

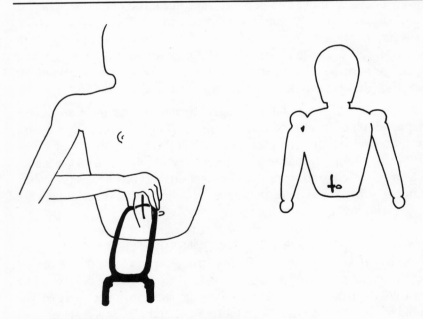

Skinfold Site 2—Abdomen (Umbilicus)
A vertical fold about one inch to the right of the umbilicus (navel)

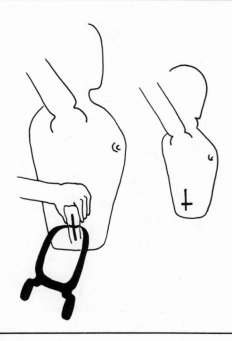

Skinfold Site 3—Hip
(Ilium)
A diagonal fold just above
the crest of the ilium

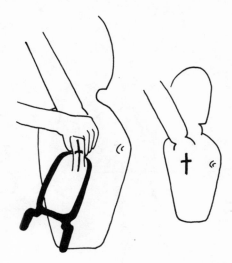

Skinfold Site 4—Side
(Axilla)
A vertical fold on the mid-
axillary line at nipple level

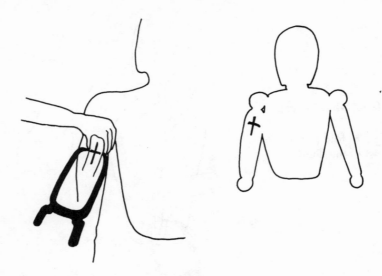

Skinfold Site 5—Arm (Tricep)
A vertical fold on the back of the upper arm midway between the shoulder and elbow joints

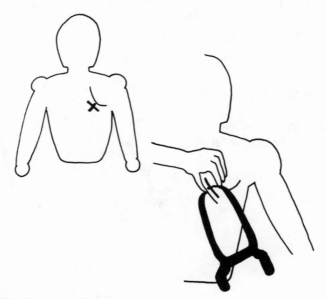

Skinfold Site 6—Back (Scapula)
A diagonal fold just below the inferior angle of the scapula

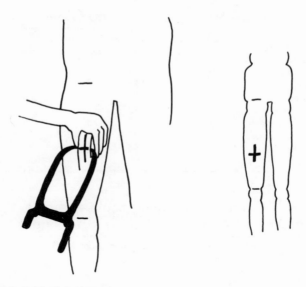

Skinfold Site 7—Thigh (Leg)
A vertical fold on the front of the thigh midway between groin line and tip
of the patella (knee)

Body Composition Rating Scale—Male
Norms—Males 35 Years and Younger

Percentage Ranking	Rating	Percent Fat	Chest mm	Abdomen mm	Ilium mm	Axilla mm	Tricep mm	Back mm	Thigh mm
95	Very Lean	6	3	4	4	4	3	4	4
85	Lean	9	7	8	6	8	6	8	6
75	Leaner Than Ave.	14	12	16	11	13	10	12	10
50	Average	18	15	21	16	17	11	15	14
30	Fatter Than Ave.	22	18	27	20	21	13	19	16
15	Fat	25	22	34	26	25	16	24	21
5	Very Fat	30	28	44	33	33	21	33	33

Norms—Males 36–45 Years

Percentage Ranking	Rating	Percent Fat	Chest mm	Abdomen mm	Ilium mm	Axilla mm	Tricep mm	Back mm	Thigh mm
95	Very Lean	8	4	6	4	4	3	4	6
85	Lean	10	8	10	8	10	7	8	8
75	Leaner Than Ave.	15	13	17	13	15	10	13	11
50	Average	19	16	22	17	19	12	17	15
30	Fatter Than Ave.	23	19	28	22	23	14	21	18
15	Fat	27	24	35	28	28	18	26	26
5	Very Fat	32	30	45	37	35	23	35	35

Norms—Males 46 Years and Older

Percentage Ranking	Rating	Percent Fat	Chest mm	Abdomen mm	Ilium mm	Axilla mm	Tricep mm	Back mm	Thigh mm
95	Very Lean	9	5	6	6	6	4	6	6
85	Lean	11	8	11	9	11	8	10	10
75	Leaner Than Ave.	16	14	18	15	17	12	15	11
50	Average	21	17	23	19	21	14	19	16
30	Fatter Than Ave.	24	20	29	23	24	16	23	19
15	Fat	29	24	36	30	30	19	28	30
5	Very Fat	34	31	46	39	36	26	38	38

Body Composition Rating Scale—Female
Norms—Females 35 Years and Younger

Percentage Ranking	Rating	Percent Fat	Chest mm	Abdomen mm	Ilium mm	Axilla mm	Tricep mm	Back mm	Thigh mm
95	Very Lean	9	5	5	4	6	5	4	5
85	Lean	14	9	8	7	11	7	6	8
75	Leaner Than Ave.	18	15	14	13	17	12	8	17
50	Average	22	18	19	16	19	15	12	24
30	Fatter Than Ave.	24	26	25	20	24	19	16	30
15	Fat	28	34	33	29	30	25	22	39
5	Very Fat	35	40	40	35	36	30	27	42

Norms—Females 36–45 Years

Percentage Ranking	Rating	Percent Fat	Chest mm	Abdomen mm	Ilium mm	Axilla mm	Tricep mm	Back mm	Thigh mm
95	Very Lean	10	6	6	5	6	6	5	6
85	Lean	16	10	8	8	12	9	8	10
75	Leaner Than Ave.	20	16	14	14	18	13	9	19
50	Average	23	18	19	18	20	17	13	25
30	Fatter Than Ave.	26	27	25	21	26	21	18	31
15	Fat	31	36	33	29	31	26	23	41
5	Very Fat	37	41	40	37	38	32	29	46

Norms—Females 46 Years and Older

Percentage Ranking	Rating	Percent Fat	Chest mm	Abdomen mm	Ilium mm	Axilla mm	Tricep mm	Back mm	Thigh mm
95	Very Lean	11	7	8	7	7	8	8	8
85	Lean	18	12	10	9	13	10	10	11
75	Leaner Than Ave.	21	18	15	16	19	15	12	21
50	Average	25	20	20	18	21	18	15	26
30	Fatter Than Ave.	30	29	26	22	27	23	20	33
15	Fat	34	37	35	32	33	27	24	43
5	Very Fat	41	42	43	39	40	34	31	48

CARDIOVASCULAR EVALUATION

Cardiovascular endurance is the ability to persist in large-muscle activities for a sustained period of time without undue fatigue. (Large-muscle activities include brisk walking, jogging, skipping rope, stair climbing, skating, and cross-country skiing.) It is the ability of the heart, blood, and blood vessels to carry oxygen to the muscle cells, to process the oxygen in those cells, and to carry off the resultant waste product.

Your heart is a muscle, and as with all muscles, exercise over a period of time can increase its size and weight. The vessels surrounding the heart also enlarge. In all, the heart becomes a stronger and more efficient organ that pumps more blood with each beat and thus needs to beat fewer times per minute to maintain proper circulation. Blood flow is improved, which in turn improves the delivery of oxygen to the muscles of the body. Consequently, fatigue from vigorous activity is delayed, and recovery from it is sooner.

The YMCA feels that the bicycle ergometer test is well suited for evaluating cardiovascular fitness, but does not recommend its use before the beginning trainee has had a complete medical examination and has been cleared by his or her physician to participate in a fitness program.

In the ergometer test the heart rate is taken while you pump the bicycle at certain speeds. The test results predict an individual's maximum working capacity and can also be used to predict maximum oxygen consumption. These measurements reflect the cardiovascular endurance of an individual, and the test is repeated during the course of a fitness program to show changes in endurance level.

Persons scoring either *fair* or *poor* in the initial ergometer test should start out more slowly in their exercise program than those scoring average or above average. "Fairs" and "poors" will probably not have the capacity to perform moderate to strenuous work and should spend several weeks walking prescribed distances and doing very simple exercises before moving up to a full-scale exercise routine. Even then, signs of overexertion should be watched for. Symptoms include dizziness and excessive redness or paleness in the face.

It is a good idea to repeat the cardiovascular/bicycle ergometer test after ten to twelve weeks into the exercise program, then again at the end of six to eight months. This will show individual progress and can also act as a spur toward greater heights of physical fitness. After the first year of training most people do not have to be tested more than once a year.

Target Weight—Males (16% Fat)

Percent Fat	Weight (pounds)																								
	120	125	130	135	140	145	150	155	160	165	170	175	180	185	190	195	200	205	210	215	220	225	230	235	240
16	120	125	130	135	140	145	150	155	160	165	170	175	180	185	190	195	200	205	210	215	220	225	230	235	240
18	117	122	127	132	137	142	146	151	156	161	166	171	176	181	186	190	195	200	205	210	215	220	225	229	234
20	114	119	124	129	133	138	143	148	152	157	162	167	171	176	181	186	190	195	200	205	210	214	219	224	229
22	111	116	121	125	130	135	139	144	149	153	158	162	167	172	176	181	186	190	195	200	204	209	214	218	223
24	109	113	118	122	127	131	136	140	145	149	154	158	163	167	172	176	181	186	190	195	199	204	208	213	217
26	106	110	115	119	123	128	132	137	141	145	150	154	159	163	167	172	176	181	185	189	194	198	203	207	211
28	103	107	111	116	120	124	129	133	137	141	146	150	154	159	163	167	171	176	180	184	189	193	197	201	208
30	100	104	108	113	117	121	125	129	133	137	142	146	150	154	158	162	167	171	175	179	183	188	192	196	200
32	97	101	105	109	113	117	121	125	129	133	138	142	146	150	154	158	162	166	170	174	178	182	186	190	194
34	94	98	102	106	110	114	118	122	126	130	134	137	141	145	149	153	157	161	165	169	173	177	181	185	189
36	91	95	99	103	107	110	114	118	122	126	130	133	137	141	145	149	152	156	160	164	168	171	175	179	183
38	89	92	96	100	103	107	111	114	118	122	125	129	133	137	140	144	148	151	155	159	162	166	170	174	177
40	86	89	93	96	100	104	107	111	114	118	121	125	129	132	136	139	143	146	150	154	157	161	164	168	173

To use, find subject's present weight at top of table, then descend vertically to horizontal row corresponding to estimated % fat; e.g., the target weight for a male who is 210 lbs. and 24% fat would be 190 lbs.

Target Weight—Female (23% fat)

Weight (pounds)

Percent Fat	105	110	115	120	125	130	135	140	145	150	155	160	165	170	175	180	185	190	195
24	104	109	114	118	123	128	133	138	143	148	153	158	163	168	173	178	183	188	192
25	102	107	112	117	122	127	131	136	141	146	151	156	161	166	170	175	180	185	190
26	101	106	111	115	120	125	130	135	139	144	149	154	159	163	168	173	178	183	187
27	100	104	109	114	119	123	128	133	137	142	147	152	156	161	166	171	175	180	185
28	98	103	108	112	117	122	126	131	136	140	145	150	154	159	164	168	173	178	182
29	97	101	106	111	115	120	124	129	134	138	143	148	152	157	161	166	171	175	180
30	95	100	105	109	114	118	123	127	132	136	141	145	150	155	159	164	168	173	177
31	94	99	103	108	112	116	121	125	130	134	139	144	149	153	157	161	166	170	175
32	93	97	102	106	110	115	119	124	129	132	137	141	146	150	155	159	163	168	172
33	91	96	100	104	109	113	117	122	126	131	135	139	144	148	152	157	161	165	170
34	90	94	99	103	107	111	116	120	124	129	133	137	141	146	150	154	159	163	167
35	89	93	97	101	106	110	114	118	122	127	131	135	139	144	148	152	156	160	165
36	87	91	96	100	104	108	112	116	121	125	129	133	137	141	145	150	154	158	162
37	86	90	94	98	102	106	110	115	119	123	127	131	135	139	143	147	151	155	160
38	85	89	93	97	101	105	109	113	117	121	125	129	133	137	141	145	149	153	157
39	83	87	91	95	99	103	107	111	115	119	123	127	131	135	139	143	147	151	154
40	82	86	90	94	97	101	105	109	113	117	121	125	129	132	136	140	144	148	152

To use, find subject's present weight at top of table, then descend vertically to horizontal row corresponding to estimated % fat; e.g., the target weight for a female who is 145 lbs. and 31% fat would be 130 lbs.

FLEXIBILITY MEASUREMENT

There is no one test that reliably determines total body flexibility, because each of our joints has specific characteristics and capabilities. However, because there is so high an incidence of low-back pain and disability among middle-aged people, and a related reduction of hip flexibility and hamstring elasticity, the YMCA recommends taking the trunk flexion test to get an idea of your general state of flexibility. As you get into your fitness program, you will discover specific joints and muscles that need special attention, and you can then begin to improve their flexibility.

The trunk flexion test is quite simple and can be taken by oneself, although some assistance would be useful. All you need is a yardstick or tape measure and a piece of adhesive tape.

THE TRUNK FLEXION TEST

Place the yardstick on the floor and the adhesive tape across it at right angles to the fifteen-inch mark (the edge of the tape closest to you is on the mark). Sit with the yardstick between your legs lengthwise and extend your legs to the tape line. Your shoes should be removed, and the heels of your feet, held about twelve inches apart, should be touching the edge of the tape (see illustration).

Keeping your fingers in contact with the yardstick, reach forward along it with both hands. Be sure your hands remain parallel—no stretching or leading with only one hand—and do not bend your knees (an assistant to keep your legs straight will help). Without jerking your body reach as far forward as you can in an effort to go farther. The stretch should be slow and gradual. To get the most indicative score, you might exhale and drop your head between your arms when reaching forward.

Your score is the most distant point on the yardstick that you reach. Take the score in inches. Make three stretches and use the farthest one

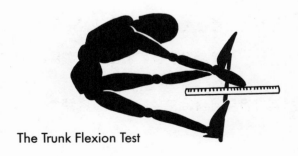

The Trunk Flexion Test

as your recorded score. You can compare your score with the following norms established by the performance of adult males and females.

Trunk Flexion Ratings

Men		Women	
Excellent	22-23 in.	Excellent	24-27 in.
Good	19-21 in.	Good	21-23 in.
Average	14-18 in.	Average	17-20 in.
Fair	12-13 in.	Fair	13-16 in.
Poor	10-11 in.	Poor	0-12 in.

MUSCULAR STRENGTH AND ENDURANCE EVALUATION

Here again there is no test that measures a person's total strength and endurance, and for the same reasons as with flexibility: no two muscle groups are quite alike, and each has different functions. Nonetheless, it is an important category, and some sort of general assessment is necessary for setting goals.

The YMCA uses push-ups, chin-ups, and sit-ups to measure strength and endurance. However, there is a bit more emphasis on timed sit-ups, which rate the strength of the abdominal muscles, the most important muscle group for middle-aged individuals. Everyone should be familiar with how to do push-ups and chin-ups, but the timed sit-ups might need some explanation.

Lie face up on the floor with your knees bent at right angles and your heels about eighteen inches from your buttocks. Clasp your hands behind your head. You want to keep your feet flush to the floor during the test, so someone to hold your feet securely in place will be a help.

With each sit-up alternately touch the inside of one knee with the opposite elbow—the left elbow to the right knee, the right elbow to the left knee. After each "up" movement return your shoulders to the floor. However, your head does not have to touch down.

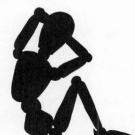

The Timed Sit-Up Test for
Muscular Endurance

Do as many sit-ups as you can within a one-minute period. Do not strain or force. The number you do is your recorded score. Compare your score with the following norms for adult men and women.

Men		Women	
Excellent	35-39	Excellent	46-54
Good	30-34	Good	35-45
Average	20-29	Average	21-34
Fair	15-19	Fair	10-20
Poor	10-14	Poor	2-9

Assuming that your tests as a whole indicate you are not up to the levels of fitness you mean to attain, you are now ready to set up a program of exercises and a schedule to reach them. At this point we want to alert you to a phenomenon in physical fitness training—retrogression.

During your first exercise sessions you will make great strides, with improvement noticeable and satisfying. But after a few weeks progress will slow down and may even stop entirely, leaving you with a sense that no further improvement is possible. This can be a discouraging time, but if you understand it is a common and normal event—and only temporary—you will work through it and continue on to your maximum level of fitness. There is rapid progression at the onset, then a slowing down that by contrast seems retrogressive, and finally another thrust upward to the top. By exercising with others at the Y you'll find support for sticking to it through those natural ups and downs.

You Can't Quit on Top

Now you must meet another challenge: staying on top of your physical condition, which means fighting off an urge to quit working out. Many people quit largely because being in good condition makes the exercises relatively easy to do and there is a feeling of no more need. However, the moment you stop exercising you also stop being physically fit. Exercise must become an integral part of your life, along with working, eating, playing. Two weeks without exercise will set you back and require easing back into your routine.

Where and When

Aside from your physical evaluations and the exercises themselves, here are some other considerations that the YMCA has found are key to setting up a program.

• *Are you self-motivated enough to exercise on your own? Or would it be better to get into a group?*

Only you can answer the first question, which then answers the second one. In any case, if you try going it alone and it doesn't work, you can always get into a group setting, which provides the structure and direction of an expert fitness counselor plus the support of the group. The latter can have a particularly salubrious effect on your attitude and your physical fitness. Harry Rock, who is with the YMCA in New London, Connecticut, has pointed out how exercise groups can have distinctly different characters:

"The A.M. group is the sleeper brigade. Everyone goes through the routines in a kind of wake-up stage, or *to* wake up. There's a lot of kidding of those who come dragging in late or don't make it one day. That's part of the challenge for this group.

"The noon group is livelier because everyone is wide awake, for one thing, but also because they are giving up most of their lunch hour and have to get back to their offices. They tend to run through the routines more quickly.

"The evening group, which meets right after work, does the routines in part as a way to wind down from their day. There's a relaxed air.

"Every group is serious about the exercises, but there is a spirit of fun all around. There are occasional luncheons, and a banquet every year where awards are given out for most miles run, most push-ups done, and so on."

• *How do you fit an exercise program into your daily schedule?*

First of all, there is no particular time of day when it is best to exercise except whenever it is convenient for you. However, you should plan on doing your exercise routine three to five times a week. It should be no fewer than three because you begin to lose conditioning after two and a half days of inactivity. Then again, if you work out more than five days a week, you are straining. Your body does need time to rest and recover.

The frequency of exercise is interrelated with the duration of each session. In order to see cardiovascular improvement, it is necessary to sustain an aerobic exercise activity for twenty to thirty minutes. But on the whole the more times a week you do exercise, the less time is needed for each session.

• *What exercises should you do?*

After taking into account any restrictions on your exercise program based on your medical examination and fitness evaluation, your program might be composed entirely of calisthenics, work on exercise machines, or athletic activity. In this book the YMCA offers a full range of choices within each category. Our advice is to choose from at least two of the three, not only to make things more interesting but to have a fully rounded program.

For instance, jogging is an excellent aerobic exercise, but it does not do much for the muscles of the arms, chest, back, or abdomen. What's more, jogging can be very stressful on the feet, ankles, and lower legs from the steady pounding. In any event, one possible combination of exercises would be calisthenics for flexibility and strength and endurance, and swimming or bicycling for cardiovascular work.

The exercises we present are designed with the average person in mind, not the serious athlete training for competition. This is not to say the latter cannot apply our offerings to his or her training.

We also include special exercises for the prevention of low-back pain, for teenagers, and for women. The YMCA has a nationally recognized healthy-back program. Local Y's lead special classes for seniors, teens, and even pregnant women.

One more thing: You must be patient. We live in an "instant society." We have come to expect most of our desires to be satisfied quickly— fast food, fast credit with a plastic card, etc. But getting yourself physically fit does not work that way. To try to get there too quickly is to risk injury and become discouraged. It takes time to do it right. The fascinating thing is, as your fitness level rises, you tend to become less and less impatient . . . about everything. Perhaps this is the result of a self-confidence born of good health.

2

Preconditioning

June is a thirty-seven-year-old mother of two who is trying to get back into the shape she was in when she got married thirteen years ago. She joined the YMCA with a friend and jumped right into an ongoing choreographed fitness class. After the first session she was so sore and stiff she was ready to quit. She noticed a tremendous shortness of breath for an hour after class and couldn't get her energy back for most of the rest of the day. Her kids found her irritable, and her husband suggested that exercise might be worse than the diets she had tried in the past.

Fortunately, when June went back to the second session, the YMCA leader talked with her before the class began. The leader suggested June do only a couple of each exercise, walk when the group jogged, and generally work at her own pace. After class the leader introduced June to the YMCA fitness director. He told June about the Y's fitness testing program and the Starter Fitness Class.

In other words, as was the case with June, it is entirely possible you are not ready to jump right into a vigorous, full-scale exercise program. It is very likely you must get into shape to begin getting into shape. This means a preconditioning program.

You will know you need preconditioning in any one or all of the following ways:

• If your physician has found you are below grade in cardiovascular efficiency; that is, if your heart is not prepared for the stress of exercise, you must precondition yourself.

• People who are obese, have high blood pressure, or suffer from orthopedic problems should precondition.

31

• You will know you are not ready to exercise full-bore when any or all of the following occur after having done some jogging, push-ups, or other fairly exertive activity:

  –you are breathing harder than you know you should.

  –your heart is beating too quickly and it takes a long time for it to regain its normal beat rate.

  –you begin feeling dizzy.

  –you feel a tightness in your chest.

  –you experience a loss of coordination.

If any of these symptoms pertain to you, you *must* begin with a preconditioning program. If you don't, you will surely get very muscle-sore at the least, and may even tear muscle tissue. You may also become seriously ill, which includes the possibility of a heart attack.

In a word, you must walk before you can run. Literally.

How to Precondition

Walking is probably the best of all preconditioning exercises, and the YMCA recommends it rather than jogging as the best way to start. Walking is a simple activity that uses many of the big muscles of the body. It also has aerobic value: it gets the blood and oxygen circulating better through the body. However, *walking must be done at a brisk pace* if it is to produce conditioning benefits.

What's "brisk"? First walk at about the speed you would use in going to an appointment, then pick up the pace. The latter will be brisk. Another indication of walking briskly is when you feel a bit of a "stitch" in your side or a slight tightening of the calf muscles after a mile or so.

Other big-muscle/aerobic-type activities you can use to precondition include stretching, jogging (once you have gotten into the program), cycling, and swimming.

Any of the exercises described in the following section on warmups and cool-downs will serve well as preconditioners. You should do the minimum number of each you choose, or even less. In all, you want to take a conservative approach. If you do jog, do not do more than a mile at first and go at a comfortable, easy pace. After a week or so you can pick up the pace and cover more distance. You can cycle at least twice as much as you jog, but again work slowly at the beginning and gradually increase your speed and distance. And swim only as much as you can without feeling deeply exhausted.

Total preconditioning time per day should be between thirty minutes and an hour. This can be spaced out over the course of your day, if convenient. For example, you might jog for fifteen minutes in the morning, do twenty minutes of calisthenics and stretching in the afternoon, and take a brisk thirty-minute walk in the evening before going to bed. Actually, this is the same sort of schedule you can use for your regular calisthenics program. It is not necessary to get all your exercise at one "sitting," so long as you get the full program done every day. If you do the whole program at once, be sure you do not overexert yourself. Take rest periods within the hour.

How Long Before "Go?"

If you have been inactive for an especially long time—a few years—and your occupation requires little or no physical exertion, the total time for preconditioning should be about six weeks; the minimum should be three weeks, no matter what.

The YMCA has worked out some parameters for determining the overall nature of a preconditioning program.

A thirty-year-old man who has been sedentary for ten years, does not smoke, is within normal weight limits, and has no known disease can probably do any program of exercises as long as he starts out slowly, exercises regularly, and makes gradual and steady progressions in the work.

A fifty-five-year-old man who has been sedentary for thirty-five years, smokes two packs of cigarettes a day, is overweight, has some history of high blood pressure, high cholesterol, and diabetes should probably have a preconditioning program that is limited to walking and rhythmic flexibility exercises.

Whatever your physical condition, common sense is the essential guideline. You can always progress upward from a low intensity of exercise. Starting at the upper limit of intensity and/or frequency is a sure way to injure yourself and also lose your enthusiasm.

You will know you are ready to "go"—ready to get into a full-scale physical fitness exercise program—when the negative symptoms described above are no longer present: you do not breathe laboriously after some jogging or push-ups, your heartbeat returns to normal within a reasonable space of time, you don't feel dizzy, you don't get a tightness in the chest, you aren't muscle-sore after a workout.

Think Fitness and Act on It

There is another sort of preconditioning we want to discuss, one that should be intrinsic to your exercise program even after you have reached your fitness-level goals. Get your *mind* into a fitness frame—think fitness even when not doing regulated exercises—and follow up with fitness-oriented activities during the day. For instance, climb or descend a couple of flights of stairs instead of taking the elevator or escalator. Climbing stairs takes fifteen times the amount of energy used for walking on the level and exercises all the muscles of the body, especially the flexors and extensors in the trunk, legs, and feet.

If you drive to your office, park in a space farthest from the entrance so you get in some walking. Get involved in participatory rather than spectator sports; join the company softball team, pull the old tennis racket out of the closet, ask a friend to play some one-on-one basketball once a week just as when you were kids.

There are other things you can do in the way of unregulated, or "unofficial," exercises while at home, at work, or anywhere else. A lot of times no one will even know what you're doing. For instance, while shaving or brushing your teeth in the morning, pull in your stomach hard and hold it in for six to ten seconds. Repeat this a few times. You can do the same thing while on the telephone, driving your car, waiting for a bus, standing around at a party. It helps keep your abdominal muscles firm.

Another exercise you can perform anywhere and at any time, while standing or sitting, is to squeeze your buttocks together and hold the pressure for a count of 10 before relaxing. Do this ten times periodically during the day. It is an excellent exercise for the lower back, having the same effect as twenty sit-ups without nearly as much exertion. Doctors recommend this exercise to waitresses and others who are on their feet a lot, as well as anyone who must sit for long periods.

Exercise Preliminaries and Warnings

HEAT ALERT

Exercising on very hot days or in very warm rooms can be dangerous. Follow the precautions and practices below when exercising under these conditions.

First, wear minimal clothing. Also be sure to replace salt that is lost through sweating. *Taking salt tablets is not advisable,* however, because of their high concentration of sodium in relation to the amount of water you're likely to consume. This can result in further dehydration of your body cells. Unless prescribed by a physician for a specific condition, such as heat cramps, salt tablets are not necessary. Instead, add more salt to the food you eat.

Because the body must have time to adapt to heat, do not exercise too strenuously during the first warm days of the hot-weather season. Being physically fit helps you to tolerate heat, but it is not a substitute for heat adaptation. The only way to increase tolerance is to exercise regularly in heat. But even then it is important to be cautious. When heat and humidity are high, either do more swimming, cut back on your other forms of exercise, or simply don't exercise at all. It is better to miss a session or two than to suffer the ill effects of working out in high heat.

A scientific standard has been developed for evaluating heat-stress danger. This temperature-humidity index (THI), which is generally reported by the Weather Bureau, can be used in judging the amount of exercise you can do at certain levels of heat.

THI	Recommendations
Below 70.0	No danger.
70.1–72.5	No sweatsuits. Overweight individuals should reduce activity.
72.6–75.0	Reduce distance and intensity of running. Overweight individuals limited to easy calisthenics and slow jogging.
75.1–77.5	Very slow jogging and light calisthenics only. Be alert for distress signs, such as getting pale or overly red in the face.
77.6–80.0	Light calisthenics. No more than a few laps of easy jogging. Swimming preferred.
Over 80.0	No gym workout. Swimming only.

OUT IN THE COLD

When exercising in the cold—running, skiing, even shoveling snow—middle-aged persons in particular should warm up adequately. It might even be best to warm up indoors. In any case, do not exercise when forced to deeply inhale excessive amounts of ice-cold air. This can result in a sudden cooling of the lower neck and chest, which may trigger reflexes causing constrictions in the heart. The constrictions may reduce oxygen supply and bring on certain kinds of heart attacks. Do not overdress to the extent that you become overheated during the exercise, and if you begin to feel warm, do not remove clothing and suddenly expose the sensitive lower neck and chest areas.

Shoveling snow, by the way, is an anaerobic, isometric-type exercise equivalent to heavy-weight lifting. It can be useful as exercise, but *only if you are physically fit* and accustomed to this kind of strenuous activity. Shoveling snow is definitely not for sedentary, unfit persons. If you do shovel snow, you should apply the same rules as mentioned above about clothing, etc., and take care that each load is not too heavy. It is better to lift a lot of small loads than a few heavy ones, especially when the snow is wet.

AIR POLLUTION AND EXERCISE

There is limited information at present on how an exercising person is affected by air pollution, but research goes on and some fairly certain things are known. For example, people do have allergic reactions to dust or specific chemicals that result in a closing of air passages; this is a potentially severe problem for asthmatics.

It has also been shown that carbon monoxide in the air reduces the transport of oxygen through the body. The heart compensates for this by beating faster. This is of particular significance to joggers, many of whom jog in city streets and along busy traffic arteries. Our advice, of course, is to jog where there is less automobile and truck traffic—or none at all, if that is possible.

EXERCISE IN HIGH ALTITUDES

The higher the altitude, the thinner the air; that is, there are fewer oxygen molecules per liter of air. You can eventually reach a height in the mountains—5,000 feet or higher—where the amount of oxygen carried by the blood is reduced to the extent that a condition called *hypoxia* develops. Under hypoxic conditions your work capacity is reduced, and any task will use a greater proportion of available oxygen. For the healthy person such effects of high altitude are annoying but not dangerous. However, for persons with a history of coronary heart disease it is wise to avoid exercise at high altitudes, since the heart's oxygen supply is already compromised.

The YMCA suggests that these persons not exercise at altitudes above 6,000 feet, which is the elevation at which airplanes are pressurized.

ON MUSCLE SORENESS

There are two types of muscle pain, or soreness, often experienced by persons who are beginning or extending an exercise program. One type, which occurs during and immediately after exercise, is apparently due to waste products formed during exercise being left in the fluids that surround the cells.

The other type of pain is a localized, delayed soreness that appears twenty-four to forty-eight hours after exercise. It is not known whether this is due to small muscle irritations or to small contractions of the particular muscles that have been used. However, this is a temporary soreness that is common when you do a new exercise or increase the intensity of those you have been doing; it will not occur once you are used to this work. If such soreness does become chronic, you must see a doctor.

To prevent muscle soreness, take a conservative approach to your exercise. Always warm up properly, and gradually increase your workload during your routines while staying within your maximum tolerance levels. And progress slowly in increasing your exercise from workout to workout. Don't overdo anything and always "cool down" after the main work with the light exercises we recommend in Chapter 4.

"NO-NO" EXERCISES

To prevent muscle soreness—or even worse effects—the YMCA feels that certain exercises should not be performed by the average person.

Avoid at all costs any bouncing and jerking exercises that force the joints to the limits of their range of motion. Indeed, you should never do any exercise at any time that puts unnatural pressures on body parts. For instance, doing exercises that put a pulling pressure on the spine and neck or place lateral pressure on a joint that does not naturally move in that direction is asking for trouble. There are plenty of other exercises available to give you the most complete workout possible without running the risk of injury.

There are seven exercises in particular to be avoided by the average person. They are: (1) the Yoga Plow, which puts unusual pressure on the neck and back; (2) the Hurdler's Stretch, for which the knees must bend unnaturally; (3) the Duck Walk and Deep Knee Bend, which puts too much pressure on the knees; (4) the Stiff-Legged Toe Touch, a traditional exercise that puts great strain on the knees and back; (5) Ballet Stretches, which should be only for trained dancers because it puts too much strain on the ligaments, knees, and lower back; (6) the Stiff-Legged Double Leg Raise, which is an old-line calisthenic that puts too much strain on the lower back; (7) the Stiff-Legged Full Sit-Up, which strains the lower back.

As a general rule, the YMCA believes that static stretching exercises such as those presented in the following chapters are most effective in preventing and relieving sore muscles while providing a sufficiently well rounded workout.

A "No-No" Exercise—Yoga Plow
It puts unusual pressure on the neck.

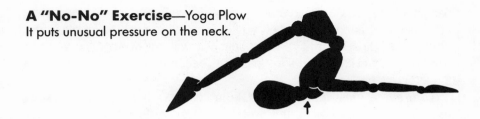

A "No-No" Exercise—Hurdler's Stretch
It puts unnatural pressure on the side of the knee.

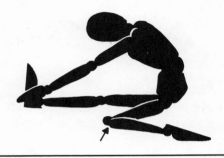

A "No-No" Exercise—Duck Walk and Deep Knee Bend
It puts too much pressure on the knees.

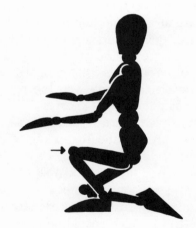

A "No-No" Exercise—Stiff-Legged Toe Touch
It puts too much strain on the back and knees.

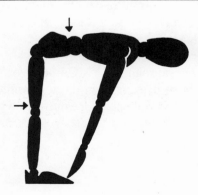

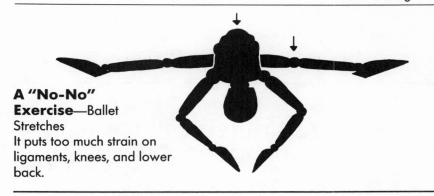

A "No-No" Exercise—Ballet Stretches

It puts too much strain on ligaments, knees, and lower back.

A "No-No" Exercise—Stiff-Legged Double Leg Raise

It puts too much strain on the lower back.

A "No-No" Exercise—Stiff-Legged Full Sit-Up

It puts too much strain on the lower back.

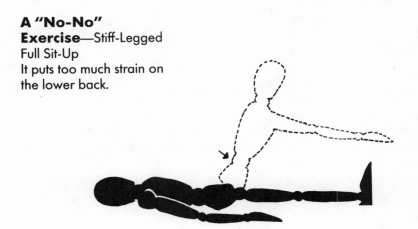

3

The Calisthenics Program—
an Overview

Tom is a CPA with a medium-sized accounting firm. As he approaches his fiftieth birthday, he can look back to over twenty years of volunteer leadership in his local YMCA. He leads the Early Bird Fitness Class three days a week and has done so longer than he cares to remember.

For Tom it is just part of living. If you start the day with enthusiasm, you'll end the day with satisfaction. He loves to welcome newcomers to his class, which is really like a club. He chats throughout the exercise routine about the importance of self-discipline and good fitness habits. His charm has made disciples of dozens of others. The early birds are a unique breed. They understand and live the principles of personal exercise.

After class most of the guys have breakfast together. Every two or three months they have a family outing. This has kept them together and reinforced their life-style over the years.

Duration, frequency, and intensity are the three principles of a progressive calisthenics program. How often, how long, and how hard should you exercise?

YMCA studies indicate that everyone should exercise a minimum of three days a week. Four or five days would be better, although changes in fitness will still occur if you work out on a three-day schedule.

Each exercise session should be for a minimum of thirty minutes, but forty-five minutes is the ideal, as this allows time for beginners to do exercises more slowly and to take fairly long rests in between. As you become more fit, the rest periods will not be as frequent or as long, but whatever their frequency or duration, they must be built into the overall schedule.

A common breakdown of time segments within a forty-five minute exercise program is ten minutes warming up, thirty minutes on cardiovascular strength and conditioning exercise, and five minutes cooling down. This breakdown is only a guide. Keep in mind that everyone is different. Each individual adapts to physical stress at his/her own rate. Feel free to adjust the daily workout schedule to your own needs and pattern. Generally, beginners take more warmup time than those in a more advanced state of fitness. Just be sure you put in the full amount of time and always warmup and cool down.

Taking Your Heart Rate

The most telling and convenient way to monitor your physical condition is to measure your heart rate. You can do it yourself. All you need is a clock with a second hand.

You don't have to take the beat of the heart itself. There are a number of pulses, or pulse points, on the body that are closer to the surface of the skin and easier to "read." Except in rare cases, the number of pulse beats per minute is equal to the number of heartbeats.

To get a heart rate, place two fingers on your chest below and to the interior side of your left nipple. You will feel your actual heartbeat. Another pulse point everyone is familiar with is on the inside of the wrist. Press your fingers lightly on the pulse point. Do not use your thumb, which tends to be less sensitive than your fingers.

Count the beat for ten seconds, then multiply the number by 6 to determine your heart rate per minute. The process takes a little practice, but should come easily after a few times.

Heart rates must be taken during the first few seconds after performing an exercise, and not beyond fifteen seconds. This is the easiest time to find a pulse, and the beat will be as close as possible to the heart rate during actual exercise.

What you are looking for is your "steady state" heart rate. That is, when a person begins exercising, the heart rate increases rapidly and continues to increase slowly for three to five minutes. It then levels off and remains steady during the remainder of the exercise. This is the "steady state."

It is generally agreed among fitness experts that to get an appreciable training effect from exercise, the workload should range from 60 to 80 percent of the individual's maximum capacity for work. This is determined by the individual's heart rate. When a person first enters into a fitness program, the *target* heart rate during exercise should be 60 percent of the predicted maximum heart rate. After the fitness level rises, the target heart rate can be increased to 70 percent, and then to 80 percent if this can be tolerated. Since heart rate decreases with age, this value becomes lower with the passing years.

The following is a scale you can use to measure, or monitor, your progress:

Age	Predicted Maximum Heart Rate	Target Heart Rate		
		60%	70%	80%
20–29	200–191	120–114	140–134	160–153
30–39	190–181	114–109	133–127	152–145
40–49	180–171	108–103	126–120	144–137
50–59	170–161	102–97	119–113	136–129

4

Warming-Up and Cooling-Down Exercises

Carol and Jim are easing into retirement—she by cutting back to twenty hours a week and he by starting a consulting business where he feels a part of the action without the pressures of full responsibility. They have been increasing their fitness activity steadily for the past two years, meeting at the Y most afternoons at about four o'clock. They engage in separate activities and then go home (or out) together for dinner.

Jim likes competition, so a good racquetball game meets his needs. Carol enjoys swimming at her own pace. The problem they both experience is the increasing evidence of bothersome little pains and strains. They recently read about the importance of stretching exercises and of warming up and cooling down. Now they spend ten minutes together in the exercise area doing the warmup stretching exercises they used to think were an unnecessary bother.

Going Up

Like a train leaving the station for a coast-to-coast trip, you must begin your daily exercise program slowly and build up a head of steam. Warmup exercises prepare the body for the heavier work to come and actually make that work easier; the train at full throttle never seems to be laboring as much as when it is getting under way. Warmup exercises prepare muscle groups and connecting tissue and get the heart and circulatory system more active.

To achieve those ends, warmups should include stretching that puts the muscles and joints through their full range of motion. For the heart and circulation you can do brisk walking, jogging, running (including

43

running in place), hops or rope-jumping, and bicycling (a stationary bike is very convenient).

The entire warmup must be done in an easy, rhythmic way, with a gradual speeding up. You start with a fox-trot, you might say, and end with a bit of swingtime that carries over to the main workout. Indeed, you might use actual music to accompany your workout from warmup right through cool-down, at least if you are exercising in private or with friends who share the same tastes in music.

Coming Down

After thirty to forty minutes of solid physical activity done at your maximum intensity, your body has gotten to running rather fast. If you stop it abruptly, the shock could prove damaging, like cold water dashed into a hot pan. To be more specific, cool-down exercises help to prevent muscle soreness by removing waste products (lactic acid) from the tissues. They also prevent dizziness, which is sometimes caused by blood "pooling" in the lower extremities. During exercise the massaging action of the muscles accommodates the increased blood flow into the muscle by speeding its removal. If exercise is suddenly stopped, the blood flow remains rapid, but there is no massaging action to remove it and blood accumulates, or pools, in the muscle. Sometimes pooling is so extensive that not enough blood is returned to the heart to maintain an effective pumping pressure. The brain and heart may be momentarily deprived of oxygen, and this can lead to fainting and dizziness; it can also induce a heart attack.

To recall our train image, you must conclude your exercise journey by easing smoothly into the station, by gradually returning your body to its nonexertive state.

The following exercises are interchangeable: you can use them for warming up and cooling down. As you will see, there is a wide variety of exercises to choose from.

For warmups the YMCA recommends that you exercise and stretch all principal body segments. Stretch and flex the neck, shoulders, trunk, hips, knees, calves, and ankles. Brisk-walk, jump rope, or jog.

For cool-downs do some mild jogging, a brisk walk, side-to-side stretches with your hands above your head, a swimmer's crawl motion while standing or walking, and some other stretching exercises.

Beginners should do the least number of repetitions specified. The more advanced your fitness, the more you do up to the maximum number.

Main Street Stroll

The basic walking exercise. Swing arms briskly and step lively with eyes forward, chest elevated, shoulders and arms relaxed. Toes and heels point straight ahead. The heel of the forward foot in every stride should strike the ground first, with the body weight carried forward and over the outer portion of the foot, then transferred to the toes.

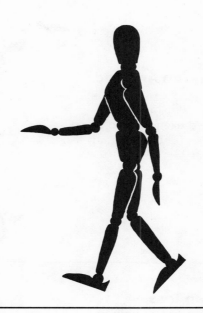

Long Strides

Same as Main Street Stroll except steps are exaggerated.

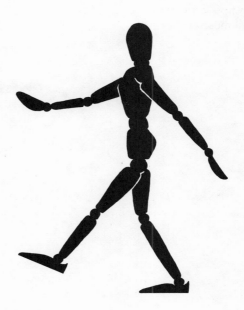

Shaking an Arm and Leg

While walking, arms and legs are shaken vigorously to stimulate circulation and relax muscles.

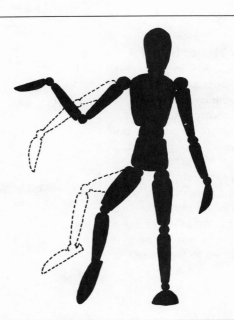

Walk on Toes

Walk on toes (i.e., balls of your feet) with good posture. Strengthens the calf muscles.

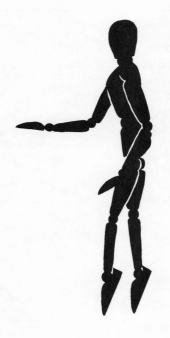

Walk on Heels

Walk erect on heels with good body posture. This should be done after walking on toes. Helps develop the muscles on the shins and stretches the calf muscles.

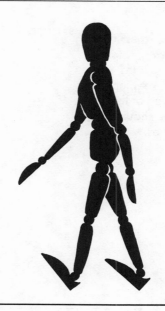

Arms High

While walking, stretch arms above shoulders and shake them easily. Helps to return the blood to the heart.

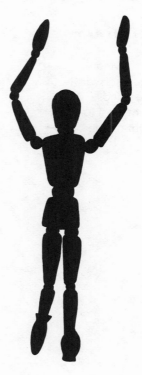

Roll Shoulders

While walking, rotate shoulders upward, back, and down, keeping the arms relaxed at the side. Relaxes the shoulder and back muscles.

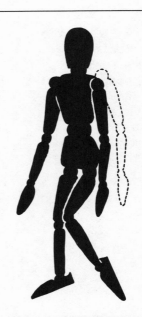

Alternate High Arm Swings

While walking, swing the arms alternately forward and back. The hands should reach at least to shoulder height on the forward swing.

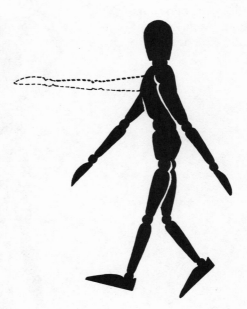

Body Bender

While walking, bend the upper torso alternately to the right and left to stretch muscles of the trunk.

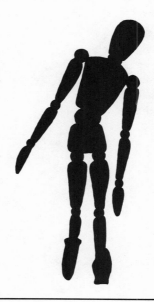

Upper Twist

While walking, twist the upper torso from side to side to improve trunk flexibility.

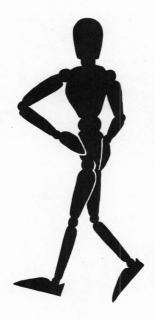

Backstroke Walk

While walking, alternately swing right and left arms upward, backward, and around to simulate swimming backstroke. Improves shoulder flexibility.

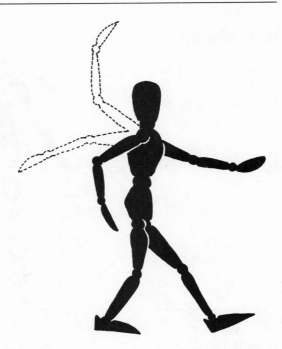

Roll Head

Roll head in circle while walking slowly to loosen up neck and improve its flexibility. Be careful not to overstrain neck structure.

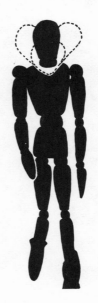

High Arm Crossovers

While walking, reach overhead and cross hands in a broad, swinging movement, then bring arms down alongside the body. Repeat as often as possible. Good for shoulder flexibility.

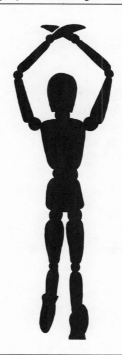

Turn Head

While walking, turn head from side to side to improve neck flexibility and relieve tension.

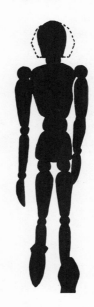

Arm Shaking
While walking, raise arms above head and shake them from side to side to aid general circulation and relax them.

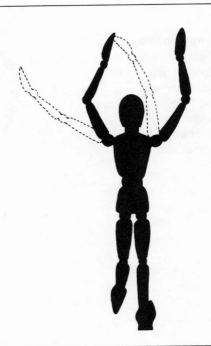

Double Arm Swing
Simultaneously swing both arms forward and back while walking. With the forward swing, the arms should come alongside your ears; backswing should take them behind your body.

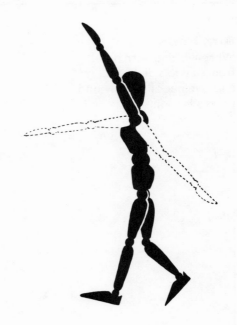

Toe-Touching

While sitting on the floor with legs extended and feet spread 6–8 inches, stretch arms and hands in front of you and bend the upper body forward. Extend hands to toes, if possible. Do not bounce to do this. Keep legs straight while reaching forward slowly and steadily. Do 10–20 forward bends.

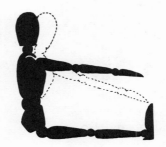

Upper Body Circles

With feet spread at shoulder width and hands held on hips, rotate upper body in a complete circle. Bend as far as you can in each direction. Do 10–20 rotations.

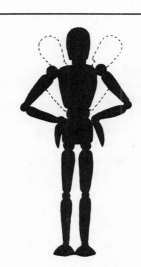

Arm Circling

While standing with feet spread at shoulder width, extend both arms fully outward and rotate them at the shoulder joints in a forward to backward direction. Do for 15–30 seconds.

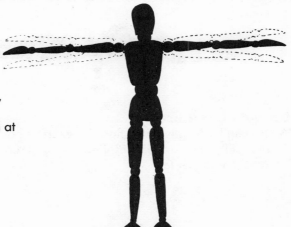

Shoulder-Joint Stretch

Stand with feet spread apart. Place the palm of each hand on your legs just below the waist. Raise the elbows to the sides. With head kept up, pull elbows backward and forward. Do for 15–30 seconds.

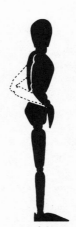

Parallel Bend

While standing with feet spread and hands set on hips, bend forward so that the upper body is parallel to the floor. Keep the head "up" at all times and do not bend the knees. Do 10–20 bends.

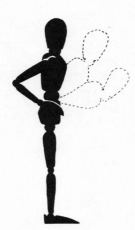

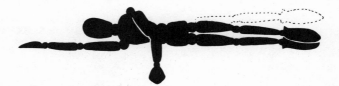

On-Side Leg Raises

While lying full length on the floor (or exercise pad), lift the top leg up and down rapidly at least 12 inches. Turn over and repeat with the other leg. Do 10–20 times per leg.

Vertical Knee Press

Stand on one foot and pull knee of the opposite leg up toward your chest with clasped hands. Raise up on toes of supporting leg when pulling the knee. Do 10–20 times with each knee.

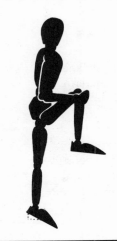

Side-to-Side Stretch

With feet spread and arms uplifted, bend the upper body from side to side as far as you can go *naturally*. Do *not* bounce body to extend stretch. This can also be done while walking. Do 10–20 times to each side.

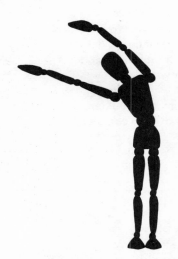

Forward-Back Bend

With hands on hips, bend forward at the waist until body is parallel to the ground. Then straighten up and bend backward as far as you can *comfortably* go. Do 10–20 times, forward and back. Helps prevent hyperextension of vertical column (spine).

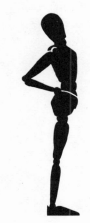

Touch Floor and Stretch

Bend forward with knees slightly flexed and touch the floor. Raise up slightly, then touch the floor again. Do 3 times. Then stretch forward and touch the floor. Each series consists of three short touches and one longer one. Do entire series 5–10 times.

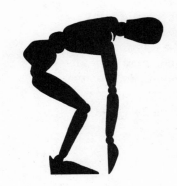

Front Crawl Stroke

This simulates the crawl stroke in swimming. While standing or walking, bend slightly forward at the waist and rotate arms in large circles from the shoulder joints. Do 30–50 complete strokes.

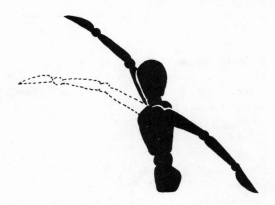

Backstroke

Stand erect and rotate arms in large circles behind you. This is the front crawl stroke in reverse. Do 30–50 complete strokes.

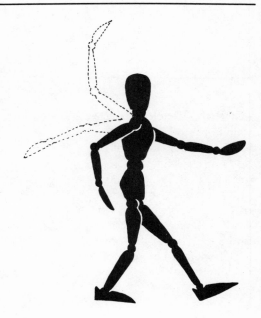

Butterfly Stroke

Bend forward slightly at the waist. Rotate both arms forward simultaneously. Do 30–50 strokes.

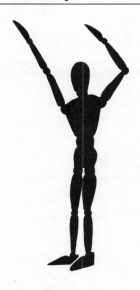

Shoulder Roll

Roll shoulders upward, back, and down, keeping arms relaxed at sides or on hips. Use only shoulders and upper back. Do 25–50 rolls. Improves shoulder flexibility and strengthens trapezius muscle.

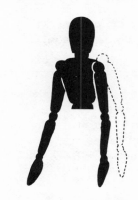

Punching Bag

Simulate punching a punching bag. Begin with arms extended, draw them back to the front of the body, then move them from left to right. The hips remain square throughout the exercise. Do 50–100 punches. Tones triceps and biceps.

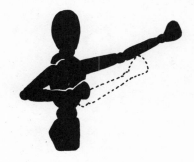

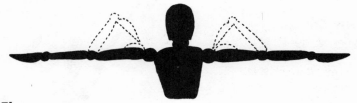

Arm Flex

Stand with feet apart, arms extended at shoulder height, palms up. Flex arms inward as "making a muscle." Then extend arms. Do 20–40 times.

Head Forward and Back

Stand with hands on hips and flex your head forward so the chin touches your chest, then extend the head backward. Be careful not to overstrain the neck structure. Do 8–12 times.

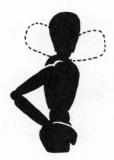

Neck Turns

Turn head to left, then right, far enough to see over each shoulder. Do 8–12 times.

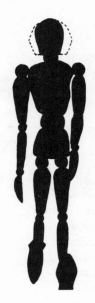

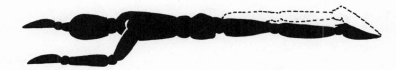

Prone Leg Raises

Lie face down on the floor. Alternately raise right and left leg 6–10 inches off the floor. Keep chest and hips touching the floor during leg raises. Do 10–20 times.

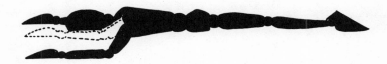

Prone Arm Raises

Lie face down on the floor. Alternately raise right and left arms about 12 inches off the floor. Keep chest and hips on the floor at all times. Do 20–40 times. Stretches chest muscles and improves shoulder flexibility.

Jumps/Hops

With feet slightly spread and hands on hips, jump about an inch off the floor. This is jumping rope without a rope. Do 20–60 times.

For variation, with each jump turn to eventually make a circle. And/or jump on one leg at a time.

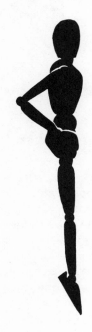

High Leg Kicks

Stand with hands on hips
and alternately kick a leg
up as high as possible.
Keep the kicking leg
straight and the supporting
leg straight as well.
Stretches muscles in back of
the leg.

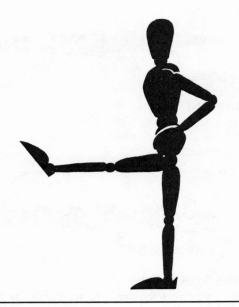

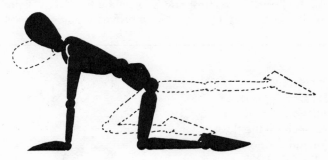

Fire Hydrant

Assume a kneeling position with hands
on the floor. Pull in your stomach to
hump your back and tuck your head
down underneath the chest as far as
possible. At the same time, bring one
leg up so the knee almost touches the
chin. Then extend this leg as far back
as possible. Bring leg in again, then
extend to the side, then return to the starting position. Do 10—20 times.
Then do the same sequence with the other leg.

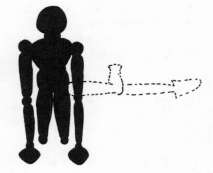

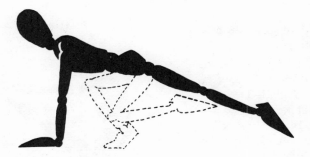

Mountain Climber

Assume a push-up position. Then bring one leg up under the chest, keeping the other leg fully extended backward and on the floor. Follow the same procedure with the opposite leg moving up under the chest. Alternate fairly rapidly to simulate crawling up an incline. Do 10–12 times with each leg. This is a good cardiovascular conditioner and it also tones up leg muscles.

Sitting Stretch

Sit on the floor with legs fully extended forward. Bend slowly at the waist and bring head down as close to knees as possible. Bend slowly forward; do not bounce to further extend. Do 10–20 times. Helps loosen hamstring muscles in back of legs.

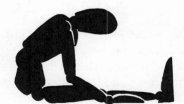

Spread Sitting Stretch

Same as Sitting Stretch except legs are comfortably spread. Bend forward at the waist to get your head as close to the floor as possible. Again, bend slowly; do not bounce to gain extension. Do 10–20 times.

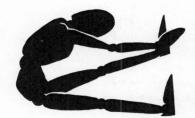

V-Seat (Advanced Exercise)

Sit on the floor with hands resting on floor at your sides or extended toward your feet. Raise legs off floor so body is resting only on your buttocks. Hold the V-Seat for a few seconds, then drop legs. Do 10–25 times.

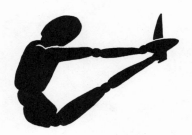

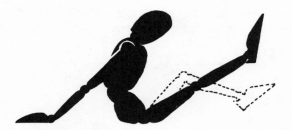

V-Seat with Flutter (Advanced Exercise)

Same as V-Seat except hands are kept palms down on the floor and legs are moved in flutter kick as they are extended. Do 20–40 kicks. Both exercises are good for abdominal and thigh muscles.

Half-Knee Bends

From a standing position bend legs to form a 90-degree angle at the knees. Heels may come off the floor. Return to starting position. Do 10–20 times. Strengthens the thigh muscles.

A variation is to make one-quarter knee bends, about 45 degrees.

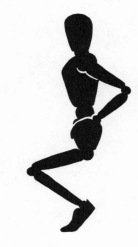

Giant Circles Forward

Stand with feet spread shoulder-width and arms extended overhead. Swing arms downward across the front of the body, then continue them up and around back to make a complete circle. Do 20–50 times. Good for shoulder flexibility.

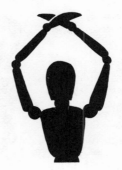

Running in Place

Run in place lifting feet at least 4 inches off the ground. To increase the work, lift the knees higher. Excellent for improving cardiovascular efficiency and also strengthens leg muscles.

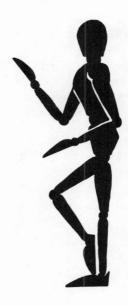

Jog

The heel, not the toes, should strike the ground first. Keep the arms relaxed, with the elbows bent at a 45-degree angle. It is important to use properly cushioned footwear and jog on ground with some cushion, if possible, rather than on pavement. Jogging stimulates the cardiovascular system, firms up leg muscles, and burns calories.

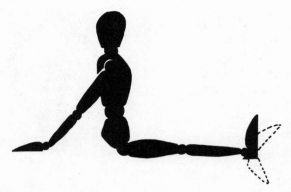

Ankle Rolls

While in a sitting position on the floor, rotate your ankles in a full circle clockwise, then counterclockwise. Continue for 30–60 seconds.

Neck Rotation

Sit on floor with legs crossed, or on a chair, and rotate your head a full 360 degrees from right to left. Do 4 times. Repeat rotation from left to right.

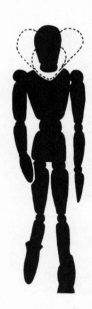

Alternate Toe Touches

From standing position, bend at the waist and touch your left foot with your right hand, then your right foot with your left hand. Remain bent over as you alternate touches and bend your knees slightly throughout the exercise. Do 10–20 times.

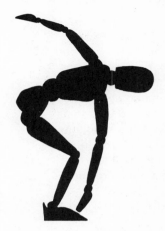

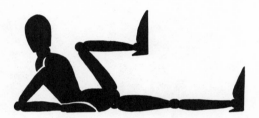

Knee Presser

Lie on the floor, your upper body raised on your elbows. Flex one knee back toward your chest and return to starting position. Do same with the other leg. Alternate for a total of 5–10 flexes per leg.

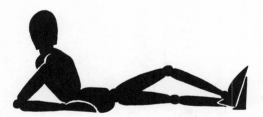

Alternate Knee Bends

Lie on the floor with the upper body raised on your elbows. Alternately flex and extend each leg while holding the heels about 4 inches off the floor, toes pointing toward the ceiling. Continue alternating for 30–60 seconds.

Push 'n' Hold

Bend over at the waist and place your hands on your knees. Pull your stomach muscles in and at the same time try to bend your trunk farther forward. Resist the trunk bend with your hands and hold for 6 seconds, then release the pressure. Repeat as often as comfortable.

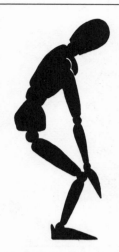

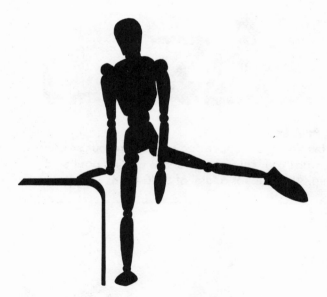

A Leg Raise

Stand beside a table or desk with fingers of the inner hand touching. Raise outside leg as high as you can, keeping the foot pointing outward at a slightly downward angle so you stretch the calf muscle. Hold at full stretch for a few seconds. Do 3–6 times. Repeat with other leg. Also good for hip muscle flexibility.

Hamstring Stretch

Stand with feet spread diagonally about 4 feet apart. Bend the left knee and concentrate your body weight over it so you feel a stretch in the right thigh. Keep your hands on top of the left knee during the exercise. Do 3–6 times. Repeat from opposite side.

Hip Flexing

Stand beside a table or desk with fingers of the inner hand just touching. Bring outer knee up as high as possible, helping it up by pulling with a hand. Keep your back straight at all times. Hold at full stretch for several seconds. Do 3–6 times. Repeat with other leg.

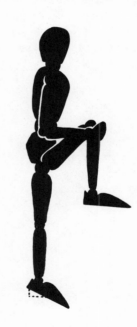

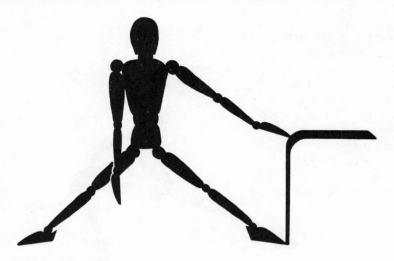

Inner Leg Stretch

Stand beside a table or desk with your near hand just touching its edge. Slide your legs apart as far as you can to stretch the insides of the thighs. Hold at full stretch for several seconds. Do 3–6 times.

Achilles' Tendon Stretch

Stand facing a wall at arm's distance. Rest your hands on the wall, then lean forward by bending your elbows and touch your head to the wall. The important thing is to keep your heels on the floor with the legs and body straight as you lean into the wall. You will feel a stretching in your calves. Hold for several seconds and return to starting position. Do 3–6 times.

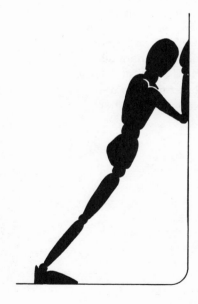

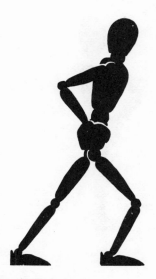
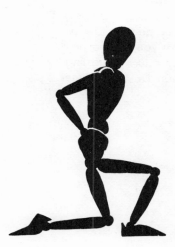

Calf/Foot Stretch

Stand in the stride position with the forward leg slightly flexed and the rear leg straight. Lean your body forward until you feel a steady stretch in the rear calf. Then flex the front knee completely, drop the rear knee almost to the floor, and roll the heel of the rear foot over its instep. Do 3–6 times. Repeat with opposite leg forward.

From a standing position, bend your left knee, and as your body lowers, raise your right leg off the ground. Do 3–6 times. Repeat with opposite leg.

Hamstring Stretch

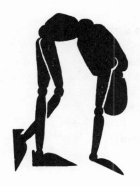

Stand and cross one leg in front of the other. Stay up on the toes of the front leg. Then slowly bend forward at the waist, keeping your rear leg straight and its heel on the floor. The front leg, of course, is slightly flexed. Bend (and stretch) until you feel the stretch in the muscles of the rear leg. Hold the position for a few seconds and return to the starting position. Do 3–6 times. Stretch the other leg in the same way. (You do not have to touch your hands to the floor during the bend. If you can, fine.)

On Your Toes

From the standing position, raise up on your toes as high as you can go, hold briefly, return to starting position. Do 10–20 times.

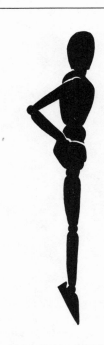

Back Stretch and Loosen

From the standing position, bend over and hold your legs just above the knees with your hands. Then, with your stomach muscles tightened, try to straighten your back while resisting it with pressure from your hands. Hold the pressure for 6 seconds, then relax. Do 5–10 times. (Of course, your hands should win the contest every time.)

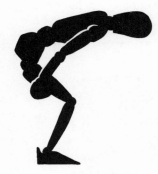

5

Flexibility Exercises

Sue was participating in a women's choreographed fitness class at the time of her first pregnancy. She was advised by many people to quit exercising altogether. But she was determined not to get out of condition despite the physical changes she knew she would be going through. The result of combined efforts by Sue, her YMCA, and her doctor and nurse was a new nationwide Y program: You and Me, Baby.

Sue found that gentle exercises could be safely done throughout pregnancy. Recovery after delivery began with simple exercises right in the hospital bed. Her postpartum routine included massage of her newborn. The key to Sue's success is steady work on strength and flexibility exercises that never strain the mother's body but help keep that body supple enough to engage in appropriate activity at a time in life when others might really slide backward.

We all marvel at the flexibility of our athletic heroes when they make wonderfully graceful movements to catch a forward pass, leap for the basket, turn the double play. We appreciate it even more as we get older because by the time we reach our mid-thirties nature has taken its course and our range of muscle and joint movement has diminished. Indeed, the diminishing begins sooner than you might think.

A newborn baby is the embodiment of pure flexibility when it—as only it can—bites its toenails. But as we age, beginning in our teens, the connective tissue (tendons and ligaments) that surrounds our joints loses some elasticity. It appears that the same thing happens to the muscles themselves. Technically, this natural deterioration is through a loss of chemical components, and nothing can be done about it any more than a tomato plant can be made to produce after its season is over.

That is why it is so important to begin flexibility exercises when you are young—fourteen years of age and up. That way the muscles, joints, tendons, and ligaments keep as much extension and elasticity as possible for a longer time.

Of course, many of you reading this book are already in your thirties and forties and have gone many years without properly exercising for flexibility. But it is not too late to recover a fair share of it, much more than you thought possible. Flexibility exercises will increase your mobility.

In a more practical vein, flexibility exercises are a major way to avoid back problems. Man's spine has not yet evolved to that point where he can or should stand upright with impunity. He must do certain things to make up for what nature has not yet provided, and flexibility exercises are the answer.

Regain your flexibility and you will work better (even if you work at a desk), you will play better, and in all, you will quit living under the shadow of imminent disaster posed by an unstretched back.

There are two kinds of flexibility exercises: *static,* characterized by a slow stretching and holding at the farthest point of the stretch, and *ballistic,* which incorporates a quick bobbing or bouncing movement. *The YMCA recommends only the static type of flexibility exercises.* We feel ballistic movement can cause unnecessary muscle soreness and pulled and torn muscles and connective tissue, because the bobbing and bouncing tend to make you extend yourself beyond your limits. You can achieve all you need in the way of flexibility with good long stretches done in a gradual way.

When doing flexibility exercises (or any other kind), *do not hold your breath* as you go through the motions. And *if a particular exercise hurts, don't do it!* You want to feel tension, but not pain!

We repeat: Always take a conservative approach to your exercise program. At the beginning do only the minimum number of repetitions and gradually work up to the maximum. If there are days when for some reason you are unable to do as many repetitions of an exercise as you did during your previous workout, so be it. Those things sometimes happen and do not necessarily mean you are going backward.

You will note that many of the exercises in this section are exactly the same as (or very similar to) those you used in your warmup and cooldown. You will simply do more of them. In fact, you will also discover that a number of flexibility exercises are repeated in the section on strength and endurance, Chapter 6. There is some overlap throughout, but this only means that with those particular exercises you get what might be called "two for the price of one."

Some of the exercises that follow are very difficult for the beginner and should not be tried until you feel you are in pretty good shape. These more difficult exercises are noted by the phrase "advanced exercise."

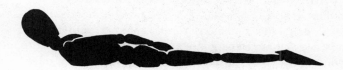

Trunk Extender

Lie face down with hands on buttocks. Raise your head and shoulders as high as possible while keeping the rest of your body on the floor. Press both hipbones into the floor. Hold momentarily, then drop head and shoulders back to the floor. Do 5–15 times. Enhances flexibility of extensor and flexor muscles of the trunk.

A variation of this exercise is to have someone hold your legs down. Then clasp your hands behind your head and raise head and shoulders.

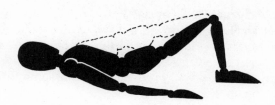

Hip Raiser (Advanced Exercise)

Lie on your back with knees bent. Lift your hips off the floor until your body straightens. Hold momentarily, then lower back to starting position. Do 5–15 times. You will feel a good stretch in your lower back and a tightening of your abdominal and buttock muscles. Be careful *not* to overarch and put excess pressure on the neck.

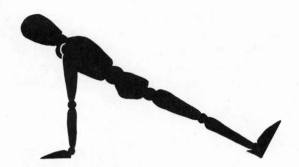

Hand and Heel Stretch (Advanced Exercise)

Take position as shown above—up on your heels, hands splayed out
behind you, entire torso off the ground. Then arch your back upward as
far as possible without forcing the upward movement. Stretches the
abdominal muscles and lower back.

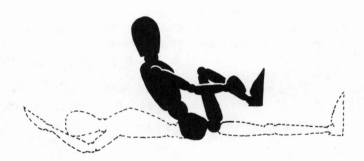

Sitting Tucks (Advanced Exercise)

Assume sitting position leaning backward slightly, your weight supported
by your buttocks. Hands are clasped across flexed knees. Then extend legs
fully, keeping them just above the floor, while placing your back flush to
the floor with arms extended backward. Return to starting position. Do 3–
6 times. Stretches the upper back muscles.

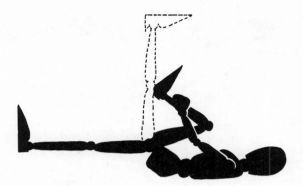

Single Leg Raises

Lie on your back and hold one knee with your hands. Lift the other leg to a vertical position and return to within 4 inches of the floor. Raise and lower leg 10–25 times. Repeat the procedure holding the other knee. Stretches muscle under the thigh (hamstring).

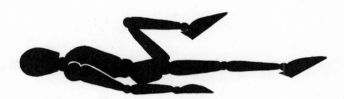

Thigh and Arch Stretch

Lie on the floor with arms at your sides, both legs extended fully and toes of both feet pointed forward. Bring your right knee back as far as possible toward the chest, then extend and slowly lower to the floor. Repeat with left leg. Keep toes of both feet pointed forward at all times. Do complete cycle 10–25 times. Stretches hamstring muscles and feet.

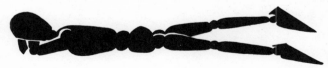

Hip Hyperextension

Lie face down on the floor, head resting on crossed arms. Stiffen right leg, then raise it off the floor from the hip. Repeat with left leg. Do with each leg 5–25 times. Always keep your stomach flat on the floor and do not rotate your pelvis when lifting your legs. Stretches hip muscles and lower back.

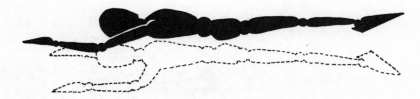

Rolling Over

Lie on your back with arms stretched above your head. Then roll your entire body to your right and onto your chest and abdomen. Reverse the roll all the way to the left until you are once again on your chest and abdomen. Roll in this way, from side to side, 6–10 times.

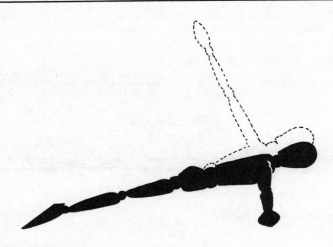

The Belly Rock

Lie on your stomach with legs fully extended and arms stretched out sideways at shoulder height. Then raise your left arm and rock your entire body to the right. (The left side of your chest will rise slightly.) Return to starting position, then raise the right arm and rock your body to the left. Do not raise your legs or pelvis during the rocking exercise. Do 5–10 times in each direction.

Twist a Hip

Lie on your back with your head resting on crossed hands, knees drawn toward your chest. Then roll your entire lower body to the left until the upper left thigh touches the floor. Keep your knees together and your feet off the floor

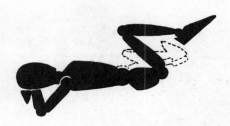

during the twist. Try to stay as flat on your back as you can, although at first this will be difficult. Return to starting position, then twist to the right. Do 5–10 times to each side.

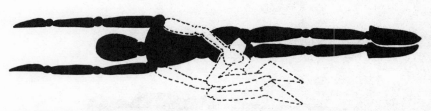

Hip Massage

Lie on your right side, your arms stretched fully overhead. Then pull both knees together up toward your chest as far as you can, using your hands to help. Return to starting position. Do 5–7 times. Repeat lying on left side.

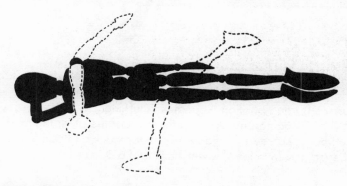

Two-Way Stretch

Lie on your right side, your head resting on your forearm. Then swing your left leg to the rear and your left arm forward. Then swing the leg forward, the arm to the rear. Swing the limbs as far as you can each time. Do 5–10 times. Repeat lying on left side.

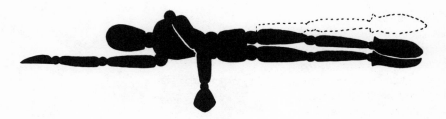

Side Leg Raises

Lie on your right side, fully extended, head resting on your right arm. Keeping the left leg straight, raise it as high as possible above horizontal, then return to starting position. Do 10—20 times. Repeat on the other side. Stretches the hip muscles.

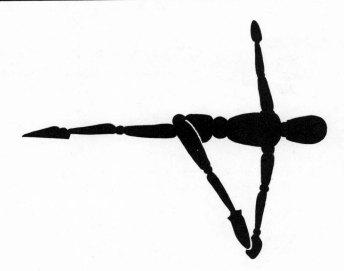

Leg-Overs

Lie on your back, arms fully extended to your sides, palms of hands facing up. Bring right leg across your body and try to touch your toes to the left hand. Return to starting position. Repeat with left leg. Do 3—10 times with each leg. When swinging one leg over, the back of the other leg must be kept on the floor; also keep shoulders, arms, and back on floor. Loosens and stretches rotator muscles of lower back and pelvic area.

Row the Boat

From sitting position on the floor, toes up, back straight, reach forward with both hands and touch your toes. Pull arms backward together as though you were rowing a boat. Do 10 times.

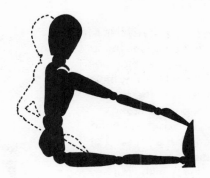

Rotation

In sitting position on the floor, with legs extended and hands placed on upper thighs, rotate your upper body to the left and swing the left arm sideways as far as you can. The right hand stays on the thigh. Return to starting position. Do 8 times. Repeat, rotating to the right.

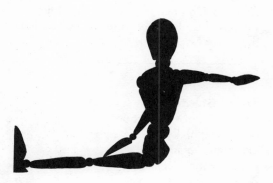

Hamstring Stretcher

Take sitting position with legs fully extended, feet spread at a 45-degree angle. Bend forward slowly at the waist and grasp the left ankle with both hands. Then stretch and try touching your head to your left knee. Resist the temptation to bounce. Hold this position for 3 seconds, then return to starting position. Repeat exercise with the other leg. Try to keep knee rigid when stretching forward, but if you can't at first, don't worry. Do 3–7 times with each leg. Stretches hamstring and lower back muscles.

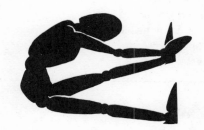

Hamstring Stretcher

Stand and cross one leg in front of the other. Stay on toes of front leg only, the foot parallel to the rear foot. Keep the rear leg straight and its heel on the floor and bend forward at the waist in a loose, relaxed way with your arms hanging down. Bend forward as far as possible 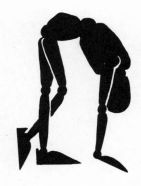 in a hanging style and hold for 20–30 seconds. Repeat with other leg forward. Do each leg exercise 2–4 times to stretch the hamstrings. This exercise has the same value as conventional toe-touching without stressing the lower back.

Sit 'n' Stretch

Sit on the floor with your back straight, legs extended but just slightly flexed, hands on knees. Bend forward and extend hands as far forward as you can above your feet. Keep your head up. Return to starting position. Do 5–15 times. Stretches lower back and hamstring muscles.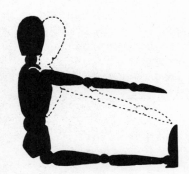

Rock 'n' Roll

Sit on the floor with knees drawn back toward your chest. Clasp hands just below kneecaps. With a slight rocking motion to begin, roll onto your upper back, then return to starting 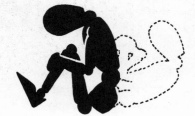 position. Do 3–10 times. Do not roll up onto your neck—that's too far. Stretches the spine and lower back muscles.

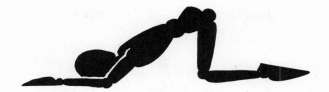

A Chest Stretcher on the Floor

Get on your hands and knees, then set your forearms flat on the floor and slowly slide them forward. Keep your back and head straight. Stretch as far forward as you can from your knees, then return to the starting position. Repeat. Do not move your chest forward with your sliding arms or you will not get the pectoral (chest) stretch intended.

A Chest Stretcher in a Chair

Sit in a chair with your hands clasped at your neck. Then bring your elbows backward as far as you can. Return to starting position and drop arms to relax for a moment. Do 5–15 times.

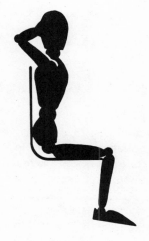

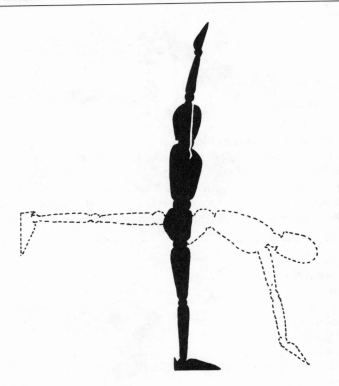

Pumping Oil

Stand with arms outstretched above your head. Lower your upper body by bending at the waist and try to touch your fingers to the floor. At the same time raise your right leg rearward as far as it will go. Return to starting position. Do 5 times. Repeat raising left leg. Be careful not to fall.

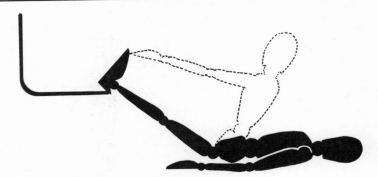

Curl-Ups (Advanced Exercise)

Lie on your back on the floor with your heels placed on the edge of a chair, arms at your sides. Slowly curl up and forward and touch your toes with your hands. Return to starting position. Do 3–10 times.

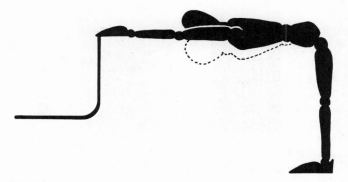

Chest Stretch

Bend forward and place your hands on the back of a chair. Keeping your back straight, push your head and chest downward with light to medium pressure. Do not try to extend lower than comfortable. Return to starting position. Do 5–15 times.

Bend 'n' Touch

Stand with feet about 18 inches apart. Keeping knees slightly flexed, touch your fingers to the floor. Return slowly to the starting position. Do 15–50 times. Stretches hamstrings and lower back.

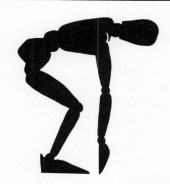

Chest Stretch

Stand with feet slightly apart and upper arms parallel to the floor. Clench fists in front of your chest, then thrust your elbows backward. Return to starting position. Do 10–30 times.

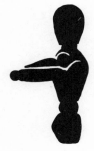

Hamstring Stretch

Stand with your hands clasped behind your back. Then, keeping your back and neck straight, slowly lower your upper body by bending at the waist. Go down as far as you can until you feel a stretching of the hamstring muscles in the back of your legs. Do 5–10 times.

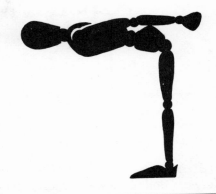

Ankle Stretcher

Stand with your hands holding a bar or the ledge of a wall, your feet about 12 inches apart. Then roll around on the outer edges of your feet. Roll to the right, then the left, 4–10 times each.

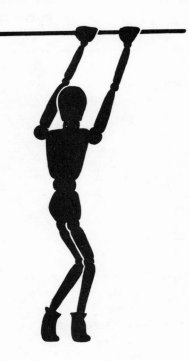

Calf Stretch

Stand with one foot about 2 feet ahead of the other in the stride position, hands clasped behind your head. Flex the forward knee, keep the rear knee straight, then lean your body forward until you feel a stretch in the rear calf. Hold for 15 seconds. Repeat with other leg forward.

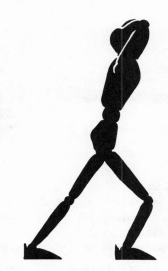

Half Squats

Stand erect with back straight, head level, and eyes looking forward. Extend arms forward and parallel to the floor. Then make a half squat by flexing knees. Keep feet slightly apart and stay up on toes, although you can also do the exercise with feet flat on the floor. Keep your back straight at all times. Do squats 5–25 times. Stretches calves and thighs.

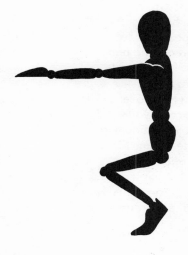

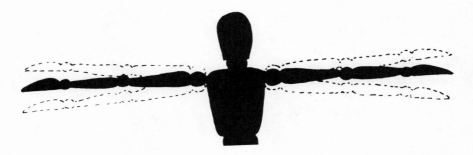

Arm Circling

Stand with feet slightly apart and arms fully extended to your sides. Rotate arms at the shoulder joints, alternating rotations from forward to backward, then backward to forward. Rotate in each direction 15–30 seconds. Exercises the deltoid muscles which cap the tops of the shoulders.

Head Rotation

While in a bent-leg standing position, feet slightly spread and hands on hips, roll your head from left to right 5–10 times, then right to left 5–10 times, to stretch your neck and relax your shoulders. You may feel some dizziness after head rotations, but this is a normal reaction, same as when you spin around in a circle.

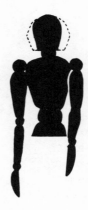

Calf Stretcher

Stand at arm's length from a wall (or any other resistant object, including an exercise partner), hands touching. Touch your head to the wall, then return to starting position. Do 5–15 times.

For variation, take the same starting position but back away from the wall while keeping your hands on it. With your feet kept flat on the floor at all times, back off until you feel a stretching of the calf muscles. Hold for several seconds.

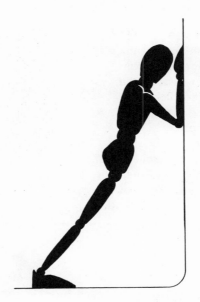

Achilles' Tendon Stretch

Stand with only the balls of your feet on the edge of a step. Extend arms forward in the air or hold on to a solid object before you. Lower heels below the step without touching them to the floor and hold for a few seconds. Then raise up on toes so heels are above them and hold for a few seconds. Do entire sequence 5–12 times.

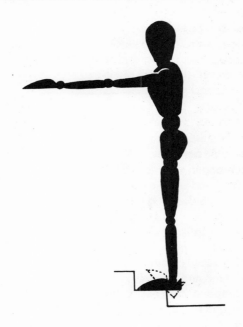

Arm Raises

Stand with arms extended at your sides, then raise them above your head. With fingers touching, stretch your arms. Return to starting position. Do 10–25 times. Loosens shoulder muscles and stretches chest. You will get an even better stretch if you touch your fingers above your head.

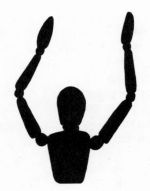

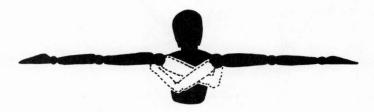

Arm Crosses

Stand with arms extended outward parallel to the floor. Cross your arms in front of your chest and return to starting position. Do 10–25 times. Stretches chest and back.

The Propeller

Stand with your feet slightly apart and arms extended at your sides. Begin to swing your arms in large sweeping circles. There are four different swing paths:

1. Arms cross in front of you moving inward, swing up above your head, then around to starting position. Do 10–20 times.

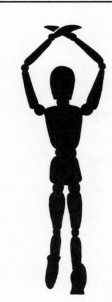

2. Arms swing outward, up above your head, then cross in front of you and back to starting position. Do 10–20 times.

3. Swing arms at each side, starting backward and swinging forward as though swimming the forward crawl stroke. Do 20–40 times.

4. Swing arms at each side, starting forward and swinging backward as though swimming the backstroke. Do 20–40 times.

In each exercise keep elbows straight (or extended) and make the widest possible circular movements. These exercises stretch all the muscles of the arms and shoulders.

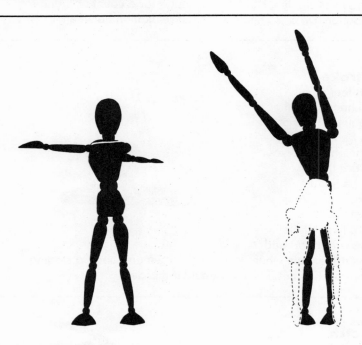

Trunk Rotation

While standing with feet shoulder-width apart, extend arms out sideways and hold at shoulder level. Then, keeping your heels flat on the floor, twist your upper body to the right as far as you can, return to starting position, and twist to the left as far as you can. Do the complete cycle, slowly, 6–12 times. Loosens and stretches back muscles and those in sides and shoulders.

Another method of trunk rotation is standing with your feet 6 inches apart, then bending forward at the waist so your arms, trunk, and head hang in a kind of loose, relaxed manner. Then twist your trunk and reach for the outside of the left foot and return to upright position. Repeat entire procedure, only try to touch the outside of your other (right) foot. Do 4–8 times for each side twist. (You may bend your knees slightly in doing this exercise, as long as you feel a stretching in the back of your legs.)

Shoulder Squeezer

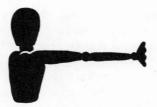

While standing, interlace fingers in front of you with palms facing outward. Arms are bent fully and held shoulder high. Then, keeping fingers interlaced, extend arms fully in front of you so elbows straighten. Hold the extension for a count of 6 and return to starting position. Do 5–15 times with brief relaxation between times.

Breaststroke

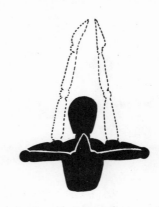

Stand with feet slightly apart and hands together palm-to-palm in front of you, arms bent and at shoulder height. Raise your arms upward then outward, the hands separating. Swing your arms down, then back to starting position. Inhale when arms are raised and thrust outward; exhale when arms swing down and back to starting position. Do 5–20 times. Loosens shoulder muscles.

Side Stretch

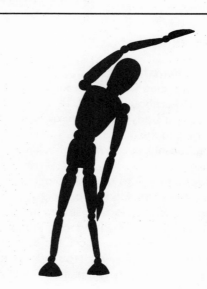

Standing with feet shoulder-width apart, extend one arm upward with palm facing inward. Extend other arm downward with the palm touching the side of your thigh. From the waist, bend to the side with the hand sliding down toward the knee. Keep the other arm extended and allow it to move with the bend of your body. Return to starting position. Repeat exercise on the other side. Alternate and do 6–12 bends on each side. Loosens and stretches lateral muscles of the body trunk.

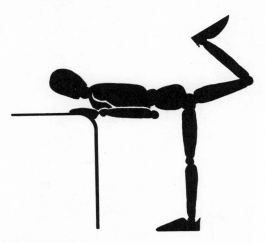

Leg-Back-Extension
Grasp edge of a sturdy table and lean over it. Bend one leg and raise it slowly behind you as high as possible with the sole of your foot facing the ceiling. Hold at farthest extension for about 6 seconds, then return to starting position. Repeat with other leg. Do with each leg 3–8 times. Exercises the hamstrings, calf and thigh muscles, and lower back. (This can be done during a private moment in your office.)

Shoulder Flex
Sit at a table (or at your desk) and put the back of each hand under the edge of it. Keeping your stomach muscles taut and your back straight, attempt to lift the table with the back of your hands. Push upward and hold for about 6 seconds, then relax. Do 3–10 times. Exercises the forearm and shoulder muscles.

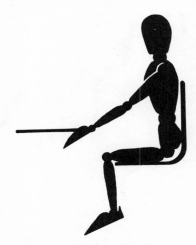

Straddle Toe-Touching

Stand with your feet about 3 feet apart and your hands clasped above your head. Then bend forward and touch your hands to the right foot. Return to upright position, then bend to touch hands to your left foot. Do 5 times for each foot.

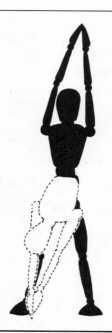

Upper Back Stretcher

Sit on a chair with your hands on your shoulders. Then try to cross your elbows in front of you. Return to starting position. Do 5–10 or more times.

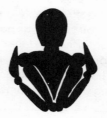

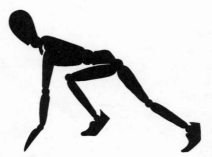

Knee and Thigh Stretch

Assume runner's starting position (as shown), but with left leg more fully extended backward. Then push right knee up toward your head. Repeat with right leg extended. Alternate and do complete cycle 5–15 times.

Shoulder Stretcher

Stand in a doorway (or sit in a chair with armrests). Touch the back of your hands to the sides of doorway. Keep your stomach muscles tight and your back straight and try to push the doorway apart. Push for about 6 seconds, then relax. Do 5–15 times. (This exercise can be performed anywhere at any time, including private moments in your office.)

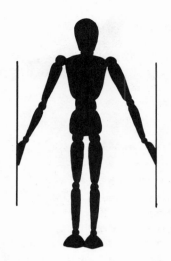

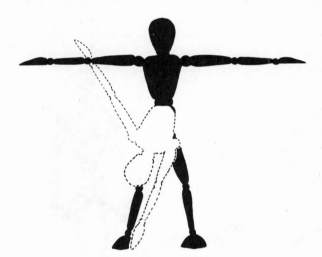

Opposite-Toe Touching

Stand with your feet apart at least shoulder-width.

Extend your arms outward at shoulder level. Bend forward at the waist and first touch your right hand to the toes of your left foot. Return to upright, then bend to touch your left hand to the toes of your right foot. Do the complete exercise 10–20 times. Stretches the hamstring, low-back extensor, and trunk rotator muscles. (If you can keep your knees straight when bending to touch the toes, fine, but if you must bend them slightly, do so. However, do not bend them so much that you feel no stretch in your rear leg muscles.)

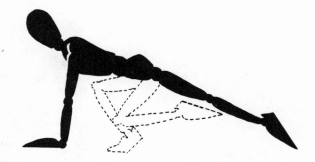

Thigh and Shin Stretcher

Assume runner's starting position (as shown), but with left leg more fully extended backward. If possible, keep the right foot flat on the floor. Push your hips down toward the floor. Hold at farthest point for a few seconds before returning to starting position. Repeat with opposite leg extended backward. Stretching should be felt in the front of the thigh on the extended leg. If not, extend that leg a bit farther backward. Do complete exercise 5–15 times.

Shoulder Stretcher

Sit in a chair and grasp it at the edges alongside your buttocks. Then try to lift the chair with both hands. Pull for about 6 seconds, then relax. Do 5–15 times. (This exercise can be performed anywhere at any time, including private moments in your office. It is excellent as a tension release.)

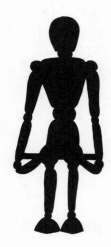

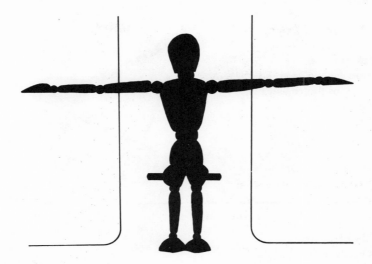

Shoulder Extension

Position yourself just outside a doorway, either sitting in a chair or standing. Extend your arms sideways at shoulder level and touch the wall with the outer edge of each hand. Push your arms backward as if trying to move the wall. Keep stomach muscles tight and head erect. Push for about 6 seconds, then relax. Do 5–15 times.

Broomstick Stretching

The following eight exercises are done with a broomstick (or other slender stick) about 42–45 inches long. All the exercises are designed to loosen muscles in neck and shoulders.

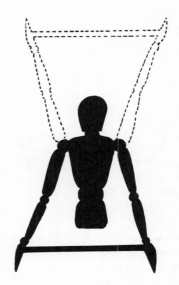

Hold stick by ends horizontally in front of your body. Keep your elbows straight. Slowly lift the stick over your head as far as possible and hold for 6 seconds. Return slowly to starting position and relax. Do 3–5 times, trying to extend the stretch a little more each time.

Hold stick by ends vertically in front of your body. Push the stick out to one side of your body while keeping the elbow of the raised arm straight. Push the stick upward as far as possible. Hold the stretch for 6 seconds. Repeat exercise on opposite side. Do 3–5 times on each side.

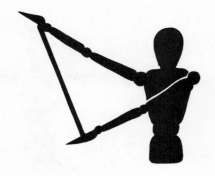

Hold stick by ends horizontally in front of the body. Tilt the stick to vertical position, move it to one side of your body, and raise it as high as possible. Keep elbow of the raised arm straight. Stretch for 6 seconds and return stick to horizontal in front of body. Repeat sequence moving stick to opposite side of body. Do 3–5 times on each side.

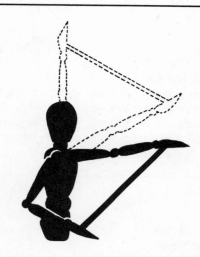

Hold stick by ends horizontally behind your body. Keeping your elbows straight, push the stick upward as high as possible. Do not bend your body forward while doing this. Stretch for 6 seconds and return to starting position. Do 3–5 times, stretching a little farther each time.

Hold stick by ends horizontally behind your back. Tilt the stick toward vertical and push it to one side of your body. Keeping the elbow of the raised arm straight, push stick upward as far as possible. Hold stretch for 6 seconds and return to starting position. Repeat on other side of your body. Do 3–5 times on each side, trying to stretch a little farther each time.

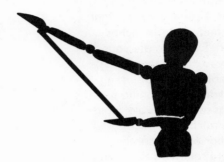

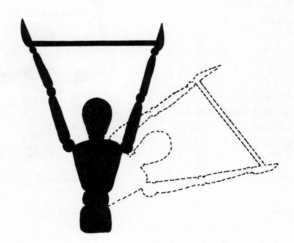

Hold stick by ends horizontally above your head. Keep your elbows straight and feet about 18 inches apart. Bend sideways as far as possible while keeping the elbows straight. Hold stretch for 6 seconds, then return to starting position. Repeat sideways bend to each side 3–5 times, stretching a little farther each time.

Hold stick by ends horizontally above your head. Keep elbows straight and feet about 18 inches apart. Slowly rotate your body to the right as far as possible, return to starting position, and rotate to the left as far as possible. Hold the stretch after each rotation for 6 seconds before returning to starting position. Do 3–5 times in each direction.

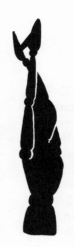

Hold stick at ends horizontally above your head. Upper arms are extended sideways; elbows are bent at 90-degree angles. Rotate the arms backward as far as possible and hold stretch for 6 seconds. Return to starting position. Do 3–5 times.

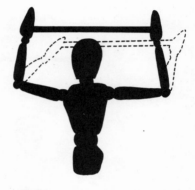

The following four exercises are good for neck flexibility and can help prevent or reduce the effects of tension headache. They can be done anywhere and at any time—in your office, at a bus stop, waiting for a traffic light, etc.

Lateral Neck Flex

Place the palm of your right hand on the right side of your head. Push head to the right and resist the push with the hand. Resist for 6 seconds, then repeat. Do the same with your left hand.

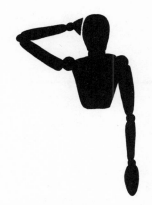

Neck Flex

Place the palms of both hands on your forehead. Push your head forward and resist this push with your hands. Resist for 6 seconds. Do 10 times. Do the exercise with your head (1) straight up, (2) flexed forward, and (3) flexed back.

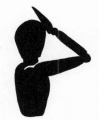

Neck Extension

Place clasped hands behind your head. Push your head backward and resist the push with your hands. Resist for 6 seconds, then repeat. Do in the same three head positions as Neck Flex.

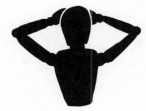

6

Strength and Endurance Exercises

John is a typical teenager. He is shy one minute and pushing the limits of everyone's tolerance the next. He has energy to burn but hates to get up before noon on school holidays.

John's body is very important to him. He wants to look good—not in terms of dress, but rather when he looks at himself in the mirror or walks onto the beach in the summer. So John goes to the Y every Saturday to work out on the machines. His goal is to build the muscles of his upper body. The weights and modern equipment are fun to work on, and he has met a number of older guys and girls who are in very good shape. The volunteer leader who staffs the exercise equipment on weekends instructs John in the importance of safety and proper technique.

Exercises to increase your strength and endurance are almost by definition harder on you than those for flexibility. Physiologically, they increase the size of muscle fiber, an action known as *hypertrophy*. The opposite action is described by a term with which you may be more familiar: *atrophy* is the decrease of muscle size through lack of use.

Muscle strength is measured by the amount of force that can be exerted by a single contraction of a muscle. *Muscle endurance* is measured by how many muscle contractions of equal power can be exerted in succession or how long a single contraction can be held.

It might seem that muscle strength is not especially important for people who do not have occupations that require lifting or pushing heavy objects and/or are not involved in leisuretime activities of a "muscular" nature. But for them—for everyone!—strong muscles are vitally important if only for one reason: they allow you to hold your body firmly upright. You cannot have good posture without muscular strength. For this reason you will find in this section a proportionally greater number of exercises meant to strengthen your abdominal muscles, for they are crucial to good posture.

Good posture, which may be generally characterized as not being round-shouldered, is not a sometime thing. Muscle strength will get you there, but to maintain it you need muscular endurance. Muscle strength and endurance are close partners in fitness.

There are certain precautions everyone must take when doing strength and endurance exercises. Because they ask more of your system than flexibility exercises do, they are potentially more dangerous.

It is advisable to do strength and endurance exercises in "sets," rather than do them continuously to the point of exhaustion. If your goal is a total of twenty push-ups, do two sets of ten each, with a rest period in between. The rest period need not be long—thirty seconds to a minute will be fine—but it is important in avoiding undue strain and possible injury.

In addition, never overstrain a particular part of the body. You might be eager to improve your abdominal muscles, and in your exuberance you may do two different exercises in a row for that area. This could create too much fatigue. What you want to do during your workout is shift forceful work from one muscle group to another and come back two or three times to the group you are most concerned about.

There is a tendency to hold one's breath during exercise routines, especially when the work is as strenuous as it is for strength and endurance. You must avoid this, for it can bring on a decreased flow of blood to the brain and result in dizziness or fainting. Whenever you hold your breath while doing heavily exertive work, there is increased pressure in the chest cavity. This pressure is transmitted through the thin walls of the large veins that return blood to the heart. The blood already in the veins is forced into the heart, which immediately pumps it out, causing a sudden increase in both blood pressure and pulse rate. As the exercise continues, there is further reduction of blood returned to the heart. With little blood to pump, blood pressure and flow suddenly decrease again. This results in decreased blood flow to the brain, resulting in dizziness and fainting. This is known as the Valsalva Effect.

As noted before, some exercises in this section on strength and endurance are also found in other calisthenics sections. The difference in this case is that for strength and endurance they are done more rapidly so you get the desired training effect.

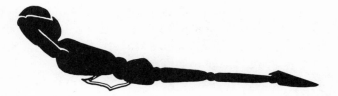

Chest Raises

Lie face down with your hands clasped behind your head. Keeping your legs on the floor, raise your entire upper body as high as possible while keeping your elbows spread wide. Return to the starting position. Do 5–15 times. Strengthens lower back, buttocks, and thighs. (You may need someone to hold your feet in place while you raise up. However, your raise will not be very high—at least at first—and you should be able to do this exercise alone.)

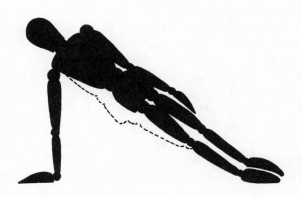

Hip Drop

Raise yourself sideways on one arm. Keeping your supporting arm and knees straight, lower your hip until it touches the floor. Return to starting position. Do 3–6 times. Repeat on other side. Strengthens side, arms, and shoulders.

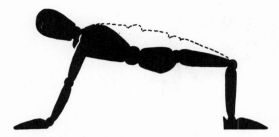

Hip Raises (Advanced Exercise)

Prop yourself face up on the floor with heels touching and knees slightly bent, the rest of your body raised and supported by your arms/hands. Then lift your midsection and let it down in a fairly rapid movement. The entire up-and-down movement should take about 6 seconds. Do 5–10 times. Do not force an upward arching of your body. Your body does not touch the floor until the exercise is concluded. Strengthens back and thigh muscles and arms.

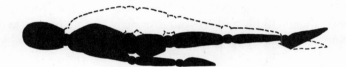

Back Arching (Advanced Exercise)

Lie on your back with your hands close to your buttocks and firmly planted. Then raise your hips off the floor as high as possible—get an arching of the back—and return to starting position.

Keep knees straight during the exercise. You will not raise very far off the floor, but will feel a stretch in the lower back and calves. Do 10–30 times in fairly rapid succession.

Strengthens lower back and buttocks.

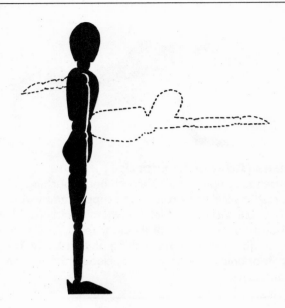

A Breaststroke

Stand with your hands at your sides. Then lower your upper body at the waist and simultaneously extend your arms fully in front of you. In a continuing motion swing your arms to the rear, then up shoulder high. Stand erect with hands at sides. Do entire cycle 10 times.

Take the Plunge

From a standing position, thrust your left leg forward a few feet and simultaneously thrust your arms out sideways at shoulder height. Return to starting position. Do 5–10 times. Repeat thrusting the right leg.

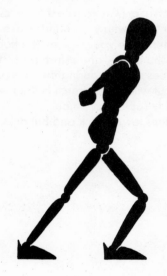

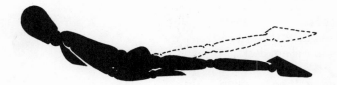

Frontal Flutter Kick

Lie on your stomach with hands tucked under your hips. Keeping your stomach on the floor, raise your chin slightly off the floor, then move your legs up and down above the floor in a flutter-kick motion. (You can bend your knees slightly if you wish.) Flutter-kick fairly rapidly for 10–20 seconds. Strengthens lower back and thighs. Caution: To prevent back injury, lift body and legs gradually. Do not raise with either a snapping or a jerking movement.

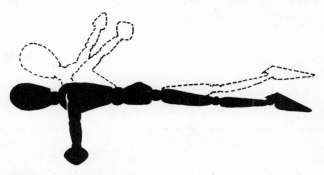

Stomach Muscle Stretcher

Lie on your stomach with arms spread fully to the sides at shoulder level. Then raise your chest, arms, and left leg off the floor. Return to starting position. Do 10 times. Repeat raising the right leg. To prevent back injury, be careful not to use snapping or jerking movements.

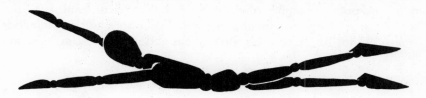

Arm and Leg Lifts

Lie face down with your arms extended over your head, legs fully extended behind. Then simultaneously raise your right arm and left leg as far as you can and hold them up for 2 or 3 seconds. Return to starting position, then raise left arm and right leg in the same manner. Alternate the action slowly; do not jerk your arms or legs. Do complete cycle 4–8 or more times. Strengthens the muscles in the back and hip.

Leg Raise

Stand beside a solidly fixed object—a railing, desk, table, etc.—with one hand on its edge. Then, keeping both legs straight, raise one leg at a time as high as possible. Keep the foot on the floor flat during the raise of the other. Return to starting position. Do with each leg 10–30 times in fairly rapid succession. Strengthens abdominal muscles and thighs. (This exercise can be done easily at home or in your office.)

For variation, hold the leg up for a few seconds with each raise before dropping it down and do fewer.

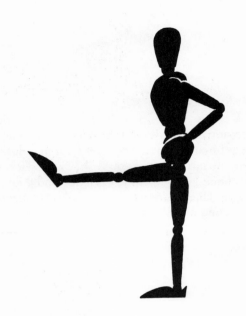

Flutter Kicks (Advanced Exercise)

Lie fully extended on your back, hands close to your buttocks. Raise your head and both legs slightly off the ground, then shake or flutter-kick your feet. Keep your legs straight at all times and your back touching the floor. Flutter-kick for 10–30 seconds. Strengthens abdominal muscles, hips, and thighs.

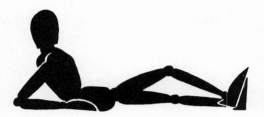

Alternate Knee-Bend Kicks

Lie on the floor in a semi-sitting position as shown, hands set close to your hips and legs fully extended. Raise both legs slightly off the floor, then bend and kick each leg alternately, keeping the opposite leg straight. You will simulate riding a bicycle. Pump legs in fairly rapid succession for 30–60 seconds. Strengthens abdominal muscles and thighs.

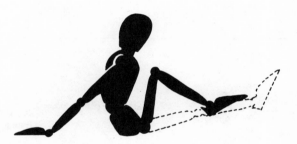

Leg Kicks (Advanced Exercise)

Sit on the floor with both knees tucked toward your chest and feet off the floor. To maintain balance, place your hands flat on the floor away from your buttocks as shown. Then thrust both legs straight out and return to starting position. Do in fairly rapid succession for 30–60 seconds. Strengthens abdominal muscles and lower back area.

Semi-Squats

Stand with hands on hips and lower body to half-squat position while thrusting arms forward. Return to starting position. Do in fairly rapid succession 10–30 or more times. Strengthens legs. (Keep head up and back straight during the entire exercise.)

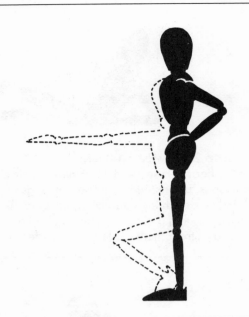

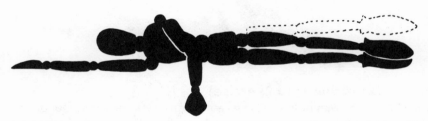

Lateral Leg Raises

Lie on one side fully extended, your head raised slightly above your arm. Keep both legs straight while raising the top one as high as possible above horizontal. Return to starting position. Do in fairly rapid succession 5–25 or more times. Repeat lying on other side. Strengthens hip muscles and thighs. As an alternative you may find it more comfortable to rest your head on your arm.

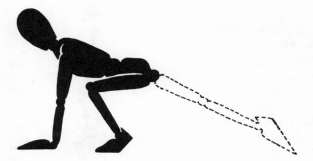

Squat 'n' Thrust (Advanced Exercise)

Starting from a standing position with your hands at your sides, four separate movements are performed in rapid succession.

1. Bend your knees and place your hands flat on the floor.
2. Thrust both legs out behind you, fully extended.
3. Return to the squat position.
4. Stand upright.

Do entire sequence 6–20 times. Strengthens muscle groups of the legs, arms, and body in general and can improve agility and quickness.

Four Hops

A series of four different hopping exercises to strengthen the calves. Do each 5–25 times before going on to the next one.

1. Hop up and down with feet together
2. Hop with legs astride.
3. Hop with legs in walking position, alternating the forward leg.
4. Hop on one leg, then the other.

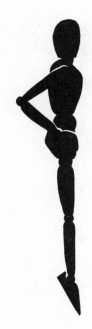

L-Hang (Advanced Exercise)

Hang fully extended from a bar using an overhand grip. Bring your legs up to a 90-degree angle and hold for 10 seconds. Return to starting position. Do 5–10 or more times. Strengthens abdomen and thighs.

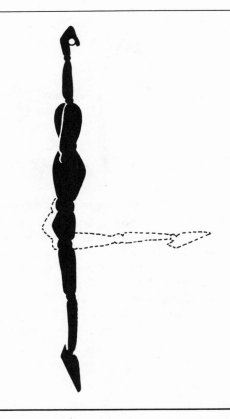

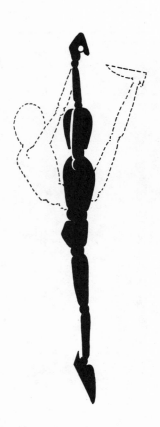

Shin-Ups (Advanced Exercise)

Hang fully extended from a bar using an overhand grip. Keep your legs straight as you bring your shins to touch the bar. Hold for 10 seconds and return to starting position. Do 3–5 or more times. Strengthens abdomen and thighs. (If you cannot reach the bar with your shins, don't fret; go as far as you can.)

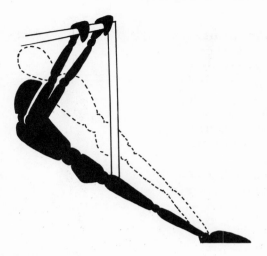

Modified Pull-Up

Grasp a bar (with palms away from you) that is about chest-high. (You will need an adjustable horizontal bar.) Then slide your feet under the bar (or along the floor) until your body and fully extended legs form a right angle to your arms. Now, holding your body firm and straight and your feet flat on the floor, pull your chest up to the bar until your chin reaches over it. Return to starting position. Do 5–25 times. Develops strength of muscles in arms, shoulders, and upper back. (This is an easier alternative to a full pull-up, while providing ample strengthening exercise.)

Pull-Ups (or "Chins")

Grasp an overhead bar that is high enough to allow you to be suspended freely from it with your arms and legs fully extended. Hold bar with palms away from you and pull yourself up until your chin clears the top of the bar, then lower yourself to starting position. Do 3–8 or more times. Develops strength and endurance of the arm muscles and the muscles in the upper back and shoulder area. As a variation, hold bar with palms toward you.

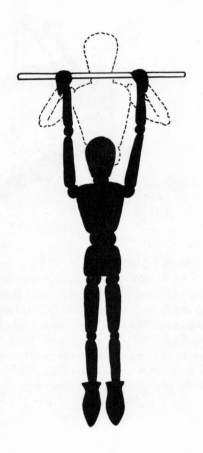

If a bar is unavailable, you can use a sturdy tree limb. Or you can hang from a doorway and raise yourself until your chin is even with your hands. You might also buy a bar with suction cups that can be set in a doorway.

Pull-Ups have traditionally been an exercise only for men, but women can and should do them also, although they may be unable to do as many. If you are unable to do even one chin, practice by hanging with arm flexed.

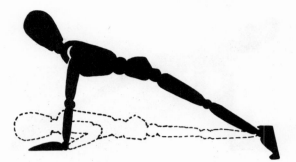

Push-Ups

The traditional Push-Up puts considerable pressure on the arms, which support most of the body's weight during the exercise. However, there are variations we present that are somewhat easier to do while giving valuable exercise.

The Traditional Push-Up

Lie on your stomach with legs fully extended and hands flat on floor at shoulder height and shoulder width apart. Your toes are touching the floor, your heels pointing straight up. Then raise your entire body by straightening your arms (remain on your toes) and lower your body to within an inch of the floor. Raise and lower your body in this manner from 3 to 15 or more times. Strengthens arm, chest, and shoulder muscles. It is important to keep your body perfectly straight during each up-and-down sequence.

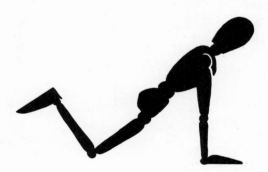

Push-Ups—A Variation

For this push-up you set your knees on the floor and raise your feet above it. The knees support your body weight, along with your arms, which are positioned in the traditional push-up manner. Raise and lower your body from the knees up in the usual manner. Do 5–15 or more times.

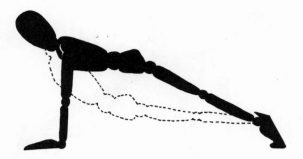

Trunk Circles

Supporting your body on hands and toes, rotate your body to the left and lower it to the floor. Raise your body, then rotate it and lower it to the right. Do 5–10 times in each direction.

Push-Ups—A Variation
Stand 3–4 feet back from the corner of a wall. Place a hand on each wall at shoulder height by leaning forward. Keep your body rigid, stomach muscles tight, and slowly lean in and touch your chin to the corner. Slowly return to the starting position. Do 5–15 or more times.

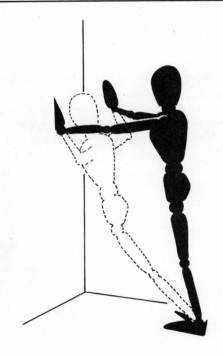

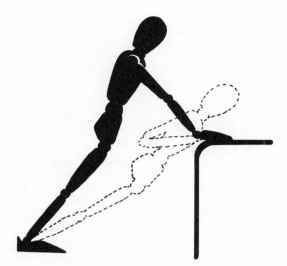

Push-Ups—A Variation
Stand 3–4 feet back from a sturdy table or desk and place hands on the edge of it. Then, keeping your body straight, lean in to touch your chin or chest to the tabletop. Return to starting position. Do 5–15 or more times.

Push-Ups—A Variation
Rest your buttocks on the edge of a sturdy table or desk with your feet about 3 feet away from it. Put your hands on the table near your buttocks. Then push your body away from the table, arching your back and pulling your head backward. Hold for a few seconds and return to starting position. Do 5–15 or more times. (This exercise also "works" your lower back muscles and is good to do periodically during the workday if you have a sedentary job.)

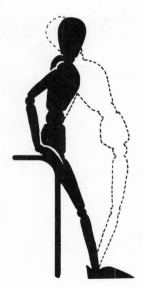

Push-Ups—A Variation
(Advanced Exercise)
Sit on an armless chair and
place your hands on the
sides at your hips. Extend
your legs outward and try
to lift your buttocks off the
seat of the chair. Hold
briefly, then lower yourself.
Do 3–5 or more times. You
probably will not rise very
much, but the exercise will
be of value nonetheless in
helping to strengthen your
arms.

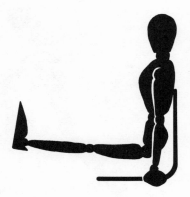

If your chair has arms, place your hands on them and lift up. You will
probably get higher off the seat. Be sure your weight is evenly distributed
on both hands or the chair may tip.

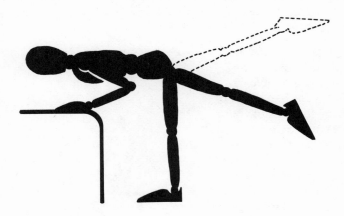

Backward Leg Raise

Lean over a table or desk as shown and slowly raise one leg as high as
possible behind you. Keep the leg straight. Return to starting position. Do
5–10 times. Repeat with other leg. Strengthens lower back muscles.

Sitting Leg Raise

Sit in a chair and hold it at the sides. Straighten both knees and raise your legs as high as you can. Return to starting position. Do 3–10 or more times. Strengthens abdominal and hip muscles.

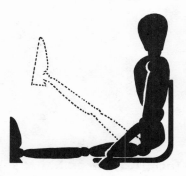

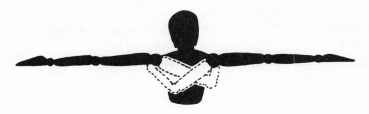

The Hug

Swing your arms across your chest and grasp your back just below your shoulders. Hold tightly and squeeze. Do 5–15 or more times. "Works" the upper back and shoulder girdle.

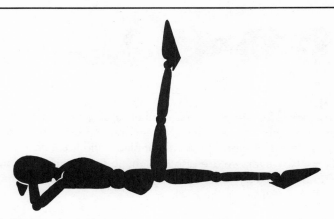

Single Leg Raises

Lie on your back with legs extended and hands clasped behind your head. Keeping your shoulders and buttocks on the floor, raise your right leg to vertical, then lower it slowly to the floor. Keep the heel of the lower leg touching the floor and both legs straight at all times. Do 5–15 or more times, then repeat with the left leg. Strengthens the hip, flexors, and abdominal muscles (and also stretches hamstrings and lower back muscles).

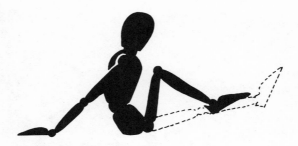

Sit 'n' Tuck (Advanced Exercise)

Sit on the floor with your hands on the floor behind your hips and both knees tucked toward your chest. Both feet are slightly off the floor. Then extend your legs straight out, keeping your feet above the floor. Return to tuck position. Do 5–20 times. Strengthens muscles in thighs, hips, and abdomen.

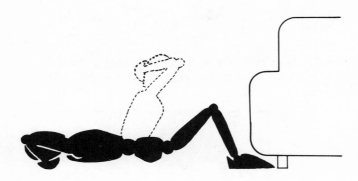

Sit-Ups

The traditional full sit-up can place a hurtful strain on the back. We therefore present it here with a warning that it is best done only by those who are already in good physical condition and have no history of back problems. However, we are also presenting some variations on the sit-up that can be just as effective for strengthening the abdominal muscles with somewhat less strain on the back.

The Traditional Sit-Up

Lie on your back with your knees bent at a 45-degree angle, your feet flat on the floor. Then, with your hands kept clasped behind your head, raise your entire upper body until it is at least vertical; you might go beyond vertical so your elbows slide past your knees. Return to the starting position. Do 5–12 or more times.

You must keep your feet flat on the floor when raising your body. If you are unable to do this, get a partner to hold your feet down or place the front half of each under a sofa or other heavy object that will serve the same purpose.

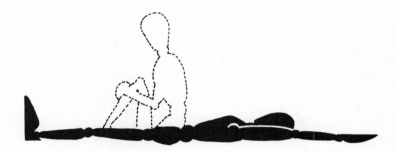

Hands-On Sit-Up

Lie fully extended on your back, legs straight, arms overhead. Curl to a sitting position while bringing your hands up to grasp your knees, which flex as you raise your upper body. Return to starting position. Do 5–20 or more times.

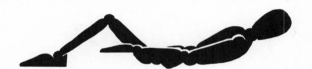

Modified Bent-Knee Sit-Up

Assume the traditional sit-up starting position except hands are placed at the sides of your thighs. Use the position of the hands as leverage to help raise your body to vertical or beyond. Do 5–12 or more times.

V-Shaped Sit-Up (Advanced Exercise)

Assume the traditional sit-up starting position. Then straighten your legs and simultaneously raise them and your upper body while thrusting your arms straight

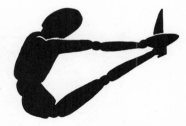

out to retain balance. Hold the resulting V-shaped position for 6 seconds, then return to starting position. Do 3–8 times.

Wrist and Forearm Strengtheners

The following three exercises, designed to strengthen the wrists and forearms, require a weighted object. This might be an old golf club with weight added to its head or a broomstick with weight attached to one end. You might also use a handgripper barbell of 5 pounds.

Abduction

Hold weighted object in one hand in front of your body, the weighted end pointing toward the floor (if using a barbell, the pointing does not apply). Then raise the weighted object with only your wrist as high as you can and slowly lower it to the starting position. Do 3–8 times with each wrist.

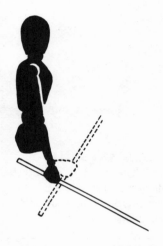

Adduction

Hold weighted object vertically at your side. Then raise it with only your wrist behind you until it reaches a horizontal position. Return it slowly to starting position. Do 3–8 times with each wrist.

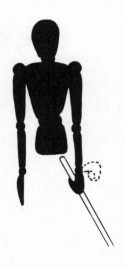

Supination and Pronation

Extend weighted object away from your body with wrist and arm straight and your arm at shoulder height. Slowly twist, using only the wrist, so the palm turns upward as far as you can twist it. Return to starting position. Then turn the palm down as far as you can and return slowly to starting position. Do 3–8 times with each hand.

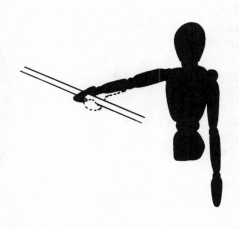

Squeeze 'n' Hold

Sit in a chair with your feet about 18 inches apart. Place the palm of your left hand on the inside of your right knee, the palm of your right hand on the inside of your left knee. Then try to squeeze your legs inward while you resist by pushing your hands outward. Hold the pressure for 6 seconds and release. Repeat as often as you like.

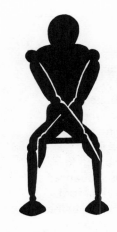

The exercise, known as abduction of the legs, strengthens the thighs, forearms, and lower back.

Push 'n' Hold

Sit in a chair with your feet spread 18 inches apart. Place the palm of your right hand on the outside of your right knee, and the palm of your left hand on the outside of your left knee. Then try to push your legs apart as you resist with your hands. Hold the pressure for 6 seconds and release. Repeat as often as you like.

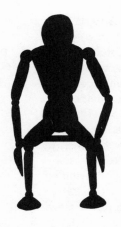

The exercise, known as abduction of the legs, strengthens the thighs, forearms, and lower back. (You can also do the exercise with your feet together.)

Step-Ups

Use a sturdy chair, stool, or bench about 12 inches high (the higher the bench, the more work done when stepping). Keeping your back straight, begin stepping onto then off the stool. Follow this sequence: step up with the right foot leading, step down with the left foot leading, step up with the left foot leading, step down with the right foot leading. This sequence is designed so the same leg does not continuously bear the burden of lifting and lowering the body.

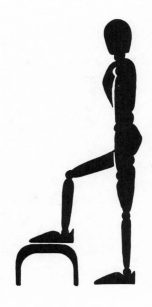

Shoulder Blade Pinch

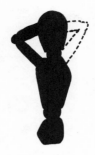

While sitting or standing, clasp your hands behind your head and point your elbows outward. Then bring your elbows forward as far as you can, touching in front of your face if possible. Then pull your elbows backward as far as you can so you feel a pinching of your shoulder blades. Return to starting position. Do complete cycle as many times as is comfortable. "Works" your shoulder blades and upper arm muscles. (Simple to do anywhere at any time, this exercise is a good way to relax after doing a lot of close work at a desk.)

Stomach Churns

Stand with feet about 1 foot apart. Lower your upper body at the waist and swing it to the left, then the center, then to the right. Return to starting position. Do 2 times. Repeat by rotating in the opposite direction. Do a total of 10–16 double revolutions per side.

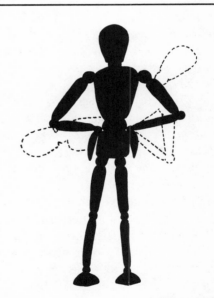

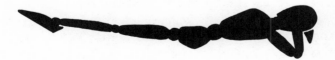

Hips Flex (Advanced Exercise)

Lie on your back, your head cradled in your hands. Raise your lower body a foot off the floor and hold for 10 seconds. Lower legs. Do 2–10 times.

7

Cardiovascular Exercises

Stan, Frank, and Guy have been running together for four years now. They meet at the Y at 5:30 three days a week without fail. They started out participating in the Fun Runs the Y organized, in which people estimate their running time for a selected distance and then win prizes for coming the closest to their projected time. In the second year they participated in three 10k runs in their area. Last year they entered as a team in a corporate challenge run.

This year they have set their goals on a half marathon that is held annually in the fall. They have developed a training schedule based on a current article in a national running magazine and have discussed it with the local Y staff. They are not sure if they are taking a step toward a future full marathon or working a bit beyond their limits.

Any vigorous activity that is sustained over a relatively long period of time is an exercise for the cardiovascular system, for it enhances the flow of blood through the system. The term for such activity is *aerobics,* a word that means "with oxygen." Oxygen produces energy needed for muscular contraction. The greater your aerobic capacity, the more oxygen you can get delivered to your body—heart, lungs, muscles— and the longer you can perform any sort of physical work.

In general, the best way to get aerobic work is through running, jogging, skiing, bicyling, swimming, choreographed exercise, and cross-country skiing. Such work means getting into a bigger exercise environment and usually blocking out more time than you would for calisthenics. Because there are going to be times when you just can't find the time or space for "major" cardiovascular activities, however, the exercises we present here will suffice as a worthwhile stopgap measure. Within a calisthenics environment, by running in place, doing jumping jacks, or jumping rope, you can get enough aerobic work to stimulate a cardiovascular response. Thus, this section is included under Calisthenics.

Some words of advice on the following activities:

When running in place, jumping rope, hopping, or doing jumping jacks, always wear proper footwear. It is time and money well spent to purchase well-made athletic shoes with sufficient cushion to keep you from injuring your feet and ankles.

Also note that fitness beginners do not have to do a lot of aerobics at a time in order to get their value. Keeping close tabs on your heart rate and other symptoms will help you know when you are exercising under more physical stress than you should be.

Running in Place

This exercise speaks for itself. You should begin at a rather slow pace for a half minute or so and gradually speed up to a comfortable limit. Overall, you should run for at least 1 minute, although as you become more fit you should be able to go for 5–20 minutes. To get a bit more work out of this exercise, you can raise your knees higher while "running."

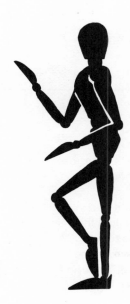

Jumping Jacks

Stand with your feet together and hands at your sides. Then, with a jump, spread your feet to a little past shoulder-width and at the same time swing your arms above your head and touch fingertips. Return to starting position. Do the sequence 10–20 or more times. The entire sequence is done in a continuing flow of motion. Each jump is executed one after the other with a rhythmic tempo. It is not necessary to do the jumps quickly, but only continually.

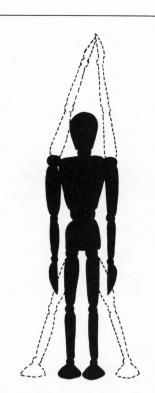

Hopping and Jumping Rope

To hop, stand with your feet slightly parted and your arms at your sides. Hold your back straight and your head erect. Maintain this posture as you begin to hop up and down on the balls of your feet. You don't need to hop very high—just enough so your feet clear the floor. Hopping steadily, you should be able to do at least 50–60 at the start of your fitness program and eventually well over 200.

For variety, with each hop you can put one foot

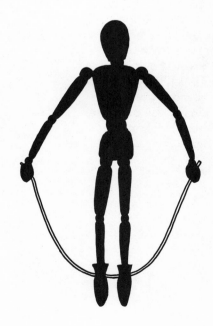

forward, the other backward. Or spread your feet to the side with one hop and bring them together with the next.

To jump rope, you maintain the same posture, and the height of your jump should also be about the same as for the hop. But of course, you will be swinging a rope over your head and beneath your feet. Get a regular jump rope, which has handles on the ends and is a bit over 9½ feet long (there are longer ones for especially tall persons). Jumping rope takes a certain kind of coordination that may take time to develop (which is also what makes it more fun than merely hopping). In any case, if you are just learning to jump rope, you probably won't be able to do more than 10–20 in succession. If so, begin the count again until you do a total of at least 75. Once you become adept, you will probably want to skip counting and jump for a particular period of time; 3–5 or more minutes will do nicely.

Step-Ups
Use a sturdy chair, stool, or bench about 9–12 inches high. (To develop cardiovascular endurance, a lower step—say, 4–6 inches high—is advised, for it permits stepping continuously for up to 20 minutes.) Keeping your back straight, begin stepping onto then off the stool and alternate the lead foot. Step up and down in a continuing rhythm—as though you were walking somewhere. As your endurance increases, you can step-up for a longer period. Begin with a minute or so and work your way up to 15 or 20 minutes. You may very well work up a little sweat with this exercise.

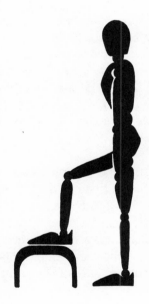

8

Lower Back Exercises

Fred has been overweight all his life. His weight was to his advantage when he played high school football, but now, at twenty-eight, he has back problems. He's in sales and constantly getting in and out of his car, carrying samples around and eating a bit too much with his customers. Every couple of months he lifts one too many boxes of sales literature and he can't move comfortably for a couple of weeks.

Last month Fred's doctor referred him to the YMCA Healthy Back program. He joined the class and feels he's making some progress. He's most impressed with the instructor, who has overcome his own back problems with steady exercise for the past four years.

A report from the United States Public Health Service some ten years ago disclosed that close to *70 million* Americans had experienced at least one incidence of severe and prolonged back pain in their lives. Another report, issued around the same time by the National Center for Health Statistics, indicated that more than 7 million Americans were being treated for chronic back pain and that 2 million more would enter into that unfortunate statistic in every subsequent year. At that rate of increase, more people may now be suffering chronic back problems than any other physical ailment.

What is really more important to understand, even if there are no statistics to support it, is that every one of us is susceptible to back problems. They can afflict people who might in every other way be perfectly healthy.

As Dr. Leon Root and Thomas Kiernan point out in their best-selling book, *Oh, My Aching Back!*, "man's Achilles' tendon is not really the cord in his heel, it is his back! The back has, for ages, been the weak

link in man's physical development. Due to its extraordinarily compli-
cated nature, plus the fact that it has been slower to structurally adjust
to man's upright position than other parts of the anatomy, the back is
more susceptible to ills than any other bodily component."

It is not all doom and gloom for the human species. If you have
already fallen into the category of low-back-pain sufferer, you can do
things to get and keep that monkey off, so to say. While chiropractic
manipulation, hot and cold packs, diathermy treatment, braces, and
other such treatments for back pain do help, they are only "Band-Aids";
the real problem does not go away for any great length of time as the
result of any such treatments. A *consistently applied* series of exercises
for the lower back is the only way to gain prolonged relief and prevent
recurrence.

These exercises are actually quite easy to do. They are not a great
strain physically. You will note that among them are exercises for the
neck and upper back. The reasoning should be obvious: these portions
of the body are intimately associated with the lower back. We have also
included exercises for excessive round-shoulderness and for building
the good posture that is essential for eliminating the excruciating pain of
a lower back gone awry.

The exercises that follow are preventive in nature. For persons who
are experiencing back problems, YMCAs offer a special course called
The Y's Way to a Healthy Back.

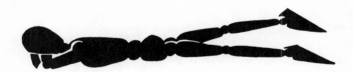

Hip Hyperextension

Lie flat on the floor and cradle your head with your arms. Stiffen your left
leg and raise it slowly from the hip. Raise and lower the leg 5–10 times.
Repeat with right leg. (Do not rotate your pelvis or raise it off the floor
when you raise your leg.)

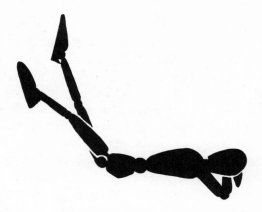

Scissors

Lie on your back with your head cradled in interlocked hands. Raise your legs in the air as vertically as you can and crisscross them in the manner of a scissors at work. Open the "scissors" as wide as you can with each "cut." Do 10 times. Then "scissors" your legs from front to back, again opening them as wide as possible. Do 10 times. Be sure to keep your back and hips flat on the floor throughout the exercise.

Knee-Nose Touch

Lie fully extended on your back, then bring your left knee back toward your chest with both hands. At the same time, raise and bring your head forward and "kiss" the knee. Hold the "kiss" for 5 seconds. Drop only your head back briefly, then raise it again to "kiss" the knee. Do the cycle 5 times. Repeat with your right knee raised. When you raise the one leg, extend the other so it stays on the floor.

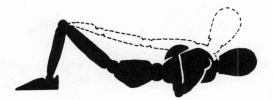

Half Sit-Ups

Lie on your back with your hands across your chest, your knees bent as shown. Then, raising only your head and shoulders, reach out and touch the top of your knees with your hands. Hold this position for 5 seconds, then return to starting position. Do 5–10 times. This exercise does the work of a traditional sit-up in strengthening abdomen and lower back muscles, but without causing back strain.

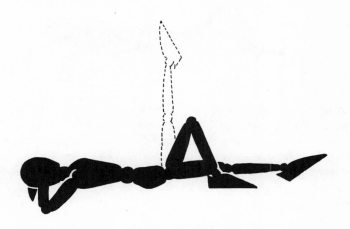

Single Leg Raises

Lie on your back with your head cradled in crossed arms, your elbows flat on the floor. Begin with both knees bent. Then straighten the right leg so it presses flat against the floor and raise it as high as you can. At full height hold for 5 seconds, then slowly lower the leg to the floor. Do 5–10 times. Repeat with opposite leg raised. Do not *swing* your leg up—only raise it— and do not use your hands to help you. Keep your lower back flat on the floor throughout.

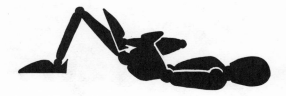

Knee Raises

Lie on your back with both knees raised. Then, with both hands, pull the right knee back toward your chest as far as you can. Hold for 5 seconds, then return to starting position. Do 5–10 times. Repeat with the left knee. Then pull both knees back at the same time. Do 5–10 times. Keep your head and shoulders on the floor throughout exercises.

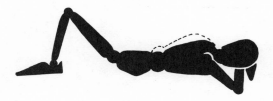

Pelvic Tilt

While lying on your back with your head cradled in crossed arms, contract the muscles of your buttocks. Clench them for a count of 5, then relax. Do 5–10 times. Keep your spine flat against the floor at all times. Do not attempt to flatten your spine by using your legs or abdominal muscles. Concentrate only on tightening your buttocks as hard as you can. If you squeeze hard enough, your pelvis will raise slightly and the small of your back will flatten naturally.

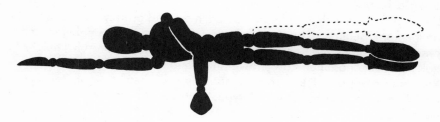

Lateral Leg Raise

Lie on your side as shown. Then raise your upper leg, keeping the knee straight. Raise the leg only 6–8 inches, and when you lower it, do not allow it to touch the bottom leg. Do 5–10 times. Repeat from other side. (As an alternative, you may find it more comfortable to rest your head on your hand.)

Hip Rotations

Lie on the floor and stretch your arms out to support your body as you draw your knees toward your chest and roll gently from side to side. Try to keep your shoulders on the floor while rolling. Roll from side to side a total of 10–20 or more times or for 30–60 seconds.

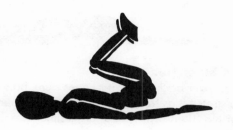

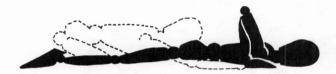

Backward Stretch

Lie face down on the floor with hands palms down at shoulder level. Then, keeping your hands and knees on the floor at all times, push your hands downward, raise your body from the knees up, and push back until your buttocks nearly touch your heels. Return to starting position. Do 5–10 times.

Body Bending

Stand with your fingers interlaced behind your head. With elbows held as shown, slowly bend your body to the right, then to the left. Return to starting position. Do for 30–60 seconds.

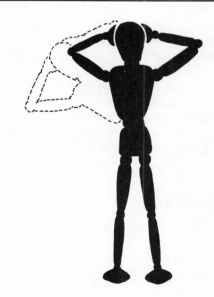

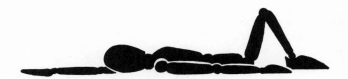

Arm Stretches

Lie on your back with your knees bent. Bring your left arm over your head and stretch it as far as you can, leaving your right arm on the floor beside your hip. Then stretch both arms simultaneously—your left arm reaching for the wall "above" your head, your right arm reaching toward your toes. Hold this stretch for a few seconds, then relax. Do 5–10 times. Repeat with the right arm over your head. Stretches the muscles in your upper back and improves the range of motion in your shoulders.

Neck Stretchers

There are three steps to this exercise, all beginning with you flat on your back and your knees raised.

1. Place the palms of your hands against the back of your head as shown and with your elbows held together bring your chin down to your chest.

2. With your hands in the same position behind your head, try to force your chin off your chest against the resistance of your hands pulling your head.

3. Keeping your chin on your chest as tightly as you can, rotate your head twice to each side.

Do the entire sequence 5–10 times. (At first you may hear some grinding or cracking of bones with this exercise, but that is not going to hurt you. You may also get a little dizzy, but that will cease as you become accustomed to the exercise.)

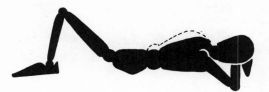

Shoulder Pinch

Lie on your back with knees raised and head cradled in crossed arms. Keep your elbows flat on the floor, then try to draw your shoulder blades together; your chest should raise slightly off the floor. Hold the stretch for a few moments, then relax. Do 5–10 times.

Sit 'n' Bend

Sit on a chair with feet apart. Bend at the waist and very loosely hang your arms between your legs, and your shoulders and head just above. Hang as low as you can for 10–20 seconds, then straighten up slowly. Do 3–5 times.

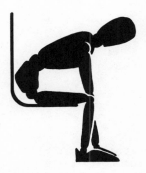

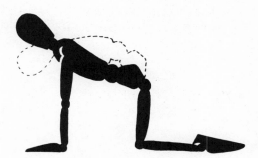

Play the Cat

Take the kneeling position as shown. Then arch your back upward like a cat, with your head dipping down. Follow this by raising your head and reversing the back action—dropping it to swayback. Do the complete cycle 5–10 times.

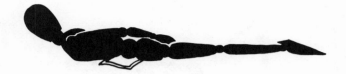

Back Arching

Lie face down on the floor with a small, firm pillow beneath your waist. Cross your hands behind your back at the waist. Then raise your head and shoulders off the floor (the rest of your body stays in place). Hold the arched position for a few moments, then slowly drop down to the starting position. Do 5–10 times. Improves posture and strengthens the shoulders and upper back muscles.

This exercise is especially recommended for young people who have round shoulders due to poor posture and suffer back pain as a result.

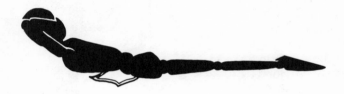

Neck-Shoulder Arching

From same position as for Back Arching, with a pillow but with hands clasped behind the head, raise neck and elbows as high off the floor as possible. Keep rest of body pressed to the floor. Hold raised position for a few moments, then slowly return to starting position. Do 5–10 times.

9

Exercises for Teenagers

Sarah is a high school student who is taking advantage of the current emphasis on women's sports. She is on the volleyball, basketball, and track teams. The summer between her freshman and sophomore years she did very little physical activity and paid for it in her fall sports. So the following summer she discovered the local Y. She got a job there working with younger children in the Day Camp program. At the end of the day she goes into the Y fitness facilities and does her own workout, toning her muscles and increasing flexibility.

It has generally been assumed that teenagers do not have to exercise simply because they are teenagers—that is, because they are flexible and active. But it is at precisely this time in life that an exercise program should be initiated. Teenagers are not, in fact, as productively active as it may seem. Their physical activity is not always of a sustained or specifically directed nature that produces or maintains good physical condition.

To begin an exercise program as a teenager is to develop a very good habit when a person is most impressionable; the habits we form when young have a tendency to stay with us throughout our lives. Moreover, exercise during youth is a form of preventive medicine, particularly with respect to reducing back problems in middle age. For the short term, the effect of exercise is good posture, which helps the teenager make a good appearance among his/her peers, for not only will the body be "standing tall" but it will look good in the latest fashions.

Because good posture is so important in the teen years as both a physical and an aesthetic plus, this special section of exercises concentrates on achieving a better carriage. As for exercises to increase

137

strength, endurance, and flexibility, those we have presented earlier in the book will apply to teenagers as well as adults. However, there are some suggestions—dos and don'ts—regarding teenage exercise that the YMCA wants to stress.

• Many young people are prone to overdo physical exercise. They do so in part because they are indeed so young and flexible and feel their "sap" with all the enthusiasm of youth. Also because of their youth they do not always understand how the body works and how much stress it can safely sustain. A further factor may be peer pressure to keep up with or do better than others as a means of acquiring social status.

There is not much the YMCA can do to change these sociocultural influences or drives, but we suggest very strongly that teenagers do warmup and cool-down exercises before and after their regular workout sessions. Warmups will help prevent serious muscle pulls and strains; cool-downs help to avoid cramps and muscle stiffness and soreness.

• The Y also suggests that teenagers wear proper footwear for their exercises. Too often young people will ignore this, which is perhaps the most important single element of equipment for good performance and injury prevention. Young people tend to wear worn-out shoes, often because it is the "in thing" among friends, or just because they are more comfortable. But athletic shoes with the heels worn down or the insteps broken out will not provide sufficient protection from the wear and tear of jogging, running, basketball, etc.

• Each teenager should find the physical activity that is most enjoyable to him or her. Exercise should be fun. If it isn't, it will not be productive, and it will be terminated—simple as that. One way to make an exercise or any physical activity more enjoyable is to find others who also enjoy it and will share the pleasure with you. There is nothing like a support group to help sustain interest in physical activity.

• The YMCA advises against wearing portable cassette players while jogging, running, or cycling. It is especially dangerous to do so in city streets or anywhere there is vehicular traffic. If you are plugged into music, you may not hear the car or truck nearby, or even be aware of it.

• Do not overeat just before an exercise session. And drink plenty of liquid when your exercise activity causes significant perspiration. The best drink is plain water, but low-calorie soft drinks are okay. In any case, the YMCA does not advise drinking liquids high in sugar content. Consider this statistic: If you run off 200 calories by way of perspiration and then drink a sixteen-ounce bottle of sugared soft drink, which contains about 280 calories, you will actually gain weight.

• The YMCA believes teenagers should avoid very heavy resistance exercises, such as power weight lifting. This is because teenagers are going through significant body changes, with musculature expanding and bones forming. Heavy-resistance exercises, which tend to put considerable strain on the maturing bones and joints, can be quite dangerous. The exercises throughout this book are at an appropriate resistive level for simple health and fitness for youths in their growing stage.

• The YMCA recommends that teenagers not jog (or run or cycle) in secluded areas. Always do so where people are nearby as a way of preventing mugging and—in the case of young women—rape.

• Girls tend to be more weight conscious than boys of the same age and should consider exercise the best form of weight control. Exercise is far safer than eating skimpy meals or missing meals altogether. Remember that every quarter mile of swimming, every mile of walking or jogging, and every four miles of cycling is one hundred calories burned.

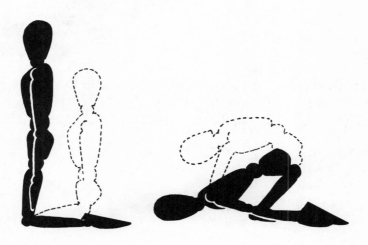

Dorsal Flat Back Exercise

Kneel on a mat and slowly lower the trunk of your body until you are sitting on your heels. Then slowly bend forward with your trunk and round your back. Slowly raise your hips, pushing your back upward, and return to starting position. Keep your head and arms relaxed during the exercise. Do several times.

Stall Bar Stretch

Begin in full standing position with hands grasping stall bars at shoulder height. Then begin walking up the bars one at a time, keeping your knees as straight as possible. Keep your hands where they are. Walk down the bars to starting position. Do 3—5 times.

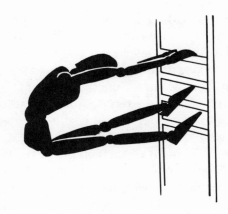

Stall Bar Forward Bend Stretch

Sit on heels facing stall bars and grasp the third or fourth rung. Bend your elbows and push the top of your head toward the bars. Press chest downward, then relax. Return to starting position. Do 5—7 times.

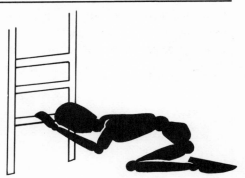

You can do this exercise and the next one at home by holding on to the seat or rung of a chair or gripping the edge of a low bureau drawer.

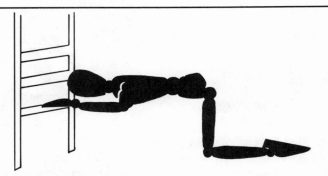

Trunk Pressing Downward

Kneel and place hands on rung of stall bars as shown. Hands should be wide apart, elbows slightly bent and pointing outward, head in line with upper body. Then contract your abdominal and buttocks muscles strongly and press your chest downward while keeping your elbows high. Slowly return to starting position. Do 3—5 times.

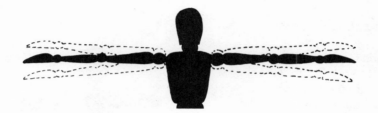

Backward Arm Circling

Sit cross-legged with your back straight and arms held out at shoulder level, palms up. Then pinch your shoulder blades together and rotate your arms backward 8–10 times. The arm circles should be slow, controlled movements with the circles small. Keep an upright posture throughout. You can do this exercise 2–3 times.

Elbow Pulling

Sit cross-legged with your back straight. Clasp your hands behind your neck and pull your elbows backward 8–10 times. You can do this exercise 2–3 times.

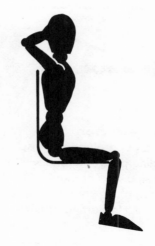

Breaking Chains

You can stand, sit, or lie supine to do this exercise. Clench your fists together in front of your chest and keep your elbows extended sideways. Then slowly pull your elbows back as if you were trying to break a chain—your hands will separate. Pull your elbows back as far as 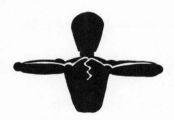 possible and hold for a few moments. Slowly return to starting position. Do 4–6 times. Keep your elbows high, and imagine great resistance when pulling elbows back.

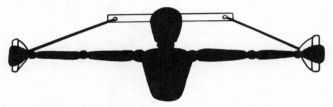

Shoulder Retractor

Sit facing the apparatus and grasp pulleys with arms extended at shoulder height, holding pulley handles with palms facing each other. Then slowly move arms sideways at shoulder level. Pinch your shoulder blades together and tighten your abdominal and buttocks muscles during the exercise. Return to starting position. Do 8–10 times. Keep your feet parallel at all times.

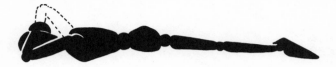

Prone Elbow Raise

Lie stretched out and face down on the floor and place your hands at the sides of your neck. Then tighten your abdominal and buttocks muscles and raise your elbows up as far as you can. Hold the position for a count of 4 and slowly lower elbows back to starting position. Do 5–10 times. Keep your legs extended and feet together throughout the exercise. As an additional exercise, you might raise your upper trunk from the floor as you raise your elbows.

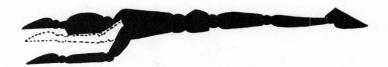

Prone Arm Lift

Lie prone on the floor with arms fully extended above your head. Then lift your arms while keeping head, trunk, and legs in contact with the floor. Slowly lower arms to floor and relax. Do 5–10 times.

Keep your pelvic girdle flush to the floor during the exercise—do not twist from side to side—and keep the body fully extended. To get full benefit of the exercise, perform the arm movements slowly.

Wall Roll-Up

Stand with your back against a wall and your heels about 4–6 inches from the wall. Then relax your upper body and bend it forward, keeping your buttocks against the wall. Bend about halfway down. Then slowly return the upper body to the starting position and extend the spine upward as much as possible without raising your heels. Return to starting position. Do entire exercise 6–8 times. Keep feet parallel throughout the exercise. Press your shoulders, back of neck, and lower back toward the 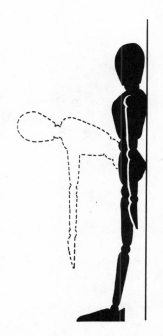 wall. Add a breathing exercise by exhaling on the forward movement and inhaling on spine extension. Another variation is to rotate your arms outward during the forward bend.

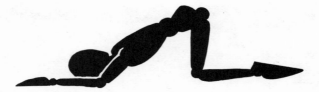

Knee Sitting Extension

Sit erect with your buttocks on your heels. Then bend your upper body forward and place your hands on the floor. Raise your hips to extend hands as far as possible. At full extension of hands, raise your chin toward the ceiling and hold for a count of 4. Then lower your head into line with the upper body, lower buttocks back to your heels, and return to starting position. Do 5–10 times. This exercise should not be done by anyone with knee problems.

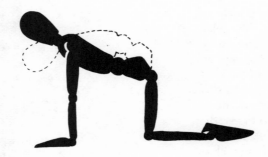

Abdominal Exercise on "All Fours"

Begin on hands and knees. Then contract abdominal and buttocks muscles and arch or hump your lower back upward; hang your head downward as you arch your back. Hold the arched position for a count of 4, then return to starting position. Do 5–10 times. Keep head level in starting position, make a strong contraction of abdominal muscles, and perform all movements slowly.

10

Exercises Especially for Women

Alice's problem is her energy level. She looks good—always has. Women in her family always kept themselves trim and dressed appropriately to the occasion. But women in Alice's family always disdained perspiration. It just wasn't proper for a lady to work up a sweat.

Alice has been active in the Y as a member of the Board, as a significant financial supporter, and when she was younger, as a member of the Youth Swim Team.

The executive director of the Y recently urged Alice to start using her locker in the women's fitness facility, and for the first time in her life she's giving it serious consideration. Maybe a little sweat wouldn't be all that bad if the result was a higher energy level.

In general, not only do women have less muscle mass than men, but the greater proportion of women's weight is lower in the body—in the pelvis, abdomen, and legs. This gives women a lower center of gravity, which enhances their balance ability, although the higher proportion of fat on the thighs can be a disadvantage in competitive running events.

But athletics aside, the distribution of fat that has been dictated by sex presents a cosmetic problem. The modern woman prefers to have a slim *total* figure. For this reason we are including the following group of exercises especially for women. The concentration is on stretching and strengthening the midtrunk and thigh areas. *These exercises will not reduce the amount of fat in these areas,* but they will tone up the muscles and give them a firmness that will leave a slimming *effect.*

Some of the exercises are for the upper body and can have the cosmetic effect of shaping women's breasts. Because women's breasts are composed of glandular and fatty tissue, exercise will not enlarge them. Heredity and total body weight determine bust size. However, exercises that tone the chest muscles under the breasts may increase overall chest girth.

We have also included four exercises recommended to relieve the discomfort of the menstrual cycle—dysmenorrhea.

Head Lifting

Lie on your back with your arms extended at your sides. Then lift only your head as high as possible and return it to starting position. Keep rest of body flat on the floor. Repeat at a steady rate, with no long pauses in between head lifts, as often as comfortable. Strengthens neck muscles.

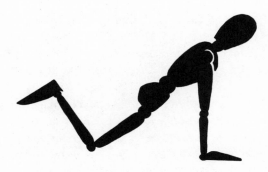

Push-Ups

Assume position as shown, supported by arms and hands and knees. Keep arms straight. Then, keeping body straight throughout, lower it to within 2–6 inches of the floor, then push yourself back up to starting position. Repeat as many times as comfortable at a steady rate. Strengthens upper arms, upper back, and shoulders.

Arm Flinging

Stand with feet apart and arms bent in front of you at shoulder level, fingers touching. Then pull or fling your elbows back behind you as far as you can, keeping your arms at shoulder level. Return to starting position. Next, straighten arms as you fling them behind you at shoulder level. Try to touch your hands. Return to starting position. Repeat, alternating the steps, as long as comfortable, using a fast pace. Strengthens shoulders, upper arms and back, and chest.

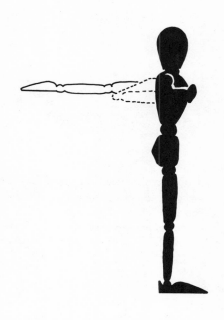

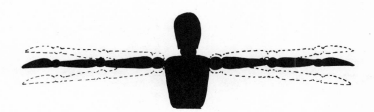

Arm Circling

Stand with feet apart and arms extended to sides at shoulder level. Then rotate your arms forward in a wide circular motion. Gradually make the circle smaller. Repeat in the opposite direction. Repeat for as long as comfortable at a steady pace. Strengthens shoulders and upper arms.

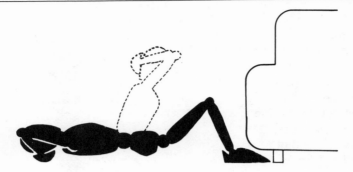

Sit-Up

Lie on your back with knees bent and feet secured either by a partner or under a solidly fixed object. Clasp your hands behind your head and raise your head so your chin touches your chest. Then curl your upper body a few inches off the ground. Return to starting position. Repeat as often as comfortable. Flattens waistline and strengthens abdominal muscles.

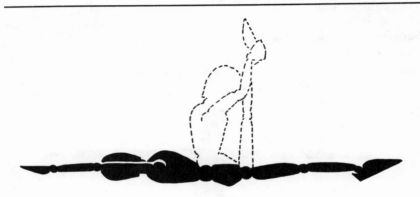

Knee-to-Nose Sit-Up

Lie on your back with your arms fully extended above your head. Then raise one leg, keeping it perfectly straight, and at the same time raise your upper body to a sit-up position. Grab the leg with your hands as close to the ankle as you can and try to touch the knee with your nose. Return to starting position. Repeat as often as you can at a steady pace. Repeat with opposite leg. Slims waistline and strengthens abdominal muscles.

Jackknife

Lie on your back with your arms fully extended above your head. Then raise both legs straight up and at the same time raise your upper body to a sitting position. Touch your toes with your fingertips while in this jackknife position. Return to starting position. Repeat as often as you can at a steady pace. Flattens waistline, strengthens abdominal muscles and lower back, and stretches hamstrings.

Spread Sit-Up

Lie on your back with arms fully extended above your head and legs spread with knees about 2 feet apart. Then raise your upper body at the waist to a sitting position and with both arms reach toward your left foot. Reach as far as you can. Return to starting position. Next, 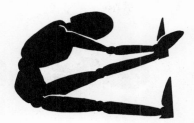 raise your upper body and reach straight forward between your legs as far as you can. Return to starting position. Next, raise up and reach toward your right foot. Repeat entire sequence as often as you can at a steady pace. Flattens waistline, strengthens abdominal muscles and back, and stretches hamstrings.

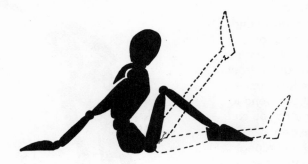

V-Sit (Advanced Exercise)

Sit on the floor with knees bent—legs close to chest, feet raised a few inches off the floor, hands palms down on floor behind you for support. Extend legs in front of you and about 3 inches off the floor. Then lift them straight up to form a "V" with your upper body, using your elbows and lower arms for support. (As you gain strength, you can use hands for support.) Return to starting position. Repeat at a steady pace as often as comfortable. Flattens waistline and strengthens abdominal and lower back muscles.

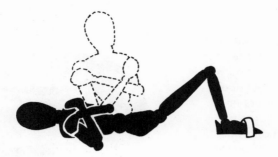

Sit-Up with a Twist

Lie on your back with knees bent, feet secured under a bed or held by a partner, your chin touching your chest and your arms folded across your chest. Then raise yourself at the waist and twist first to one side then the other while in the sit-up position. Return to starting position. Repeat as often as comfortable. Strengthens abdominal muscles and upper back.

Side Bending

Stand with feet apart and one arm bowed above your head, the other arm bowed downward in front of your body. Keep upper body straight and bend to one side as far as you can. Next, reverse arm arrangement and repeat the bending movement to the other side. Repeat as often as comfortable. Stretches lower back and strengthens hips.

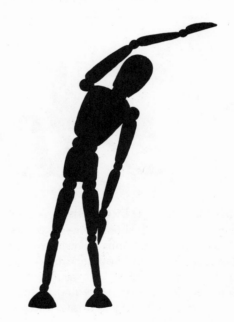

Waist Twist I

Stand with legs apart and arms bent at shoulder level with fingers not quite touching. Keeping the lower body as straight as possible, turn your upper body as far as you can to the right, then to the left. Continue twisting from side to side. Repeat as often as comfortable. Strengthens hips and lower back. You can also alternate directions from time to time.

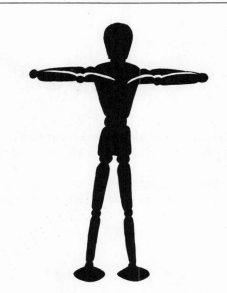

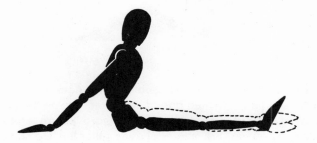

Waist Twist II

Sit on floor with legs extended straight out and toes pointing up. Place your hands palms down at your sides for support. Then roll your lower body from one side to the other, your buttocks as fulcrum. Repeat as often as comfortable. Tones and strengthens the waist, hips, and lower back.

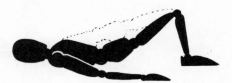

Hip Lifters (Advanced Exercise)

Lie on your back with your knees raised high and arms at your sides, with hands flat on the floor. Then lift your hips as high as you can, keeping your shoulders and feet on the floor. Return to starting position. Repeat as long as comfortable at a steady pace. Strengthens the waist, hips, lower back, and thighs.

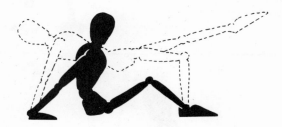

Leg Up

Take the "crab" position on the floor: seated with knees raised and hands behind you, with fingers pointed ahead. Keep feet flat on the floor. Then raise your body and extend your right leg upward. Return leg to the floor and take seated position again. Repeat using other leg. Do complete cycle as often as comfortable at a steady pace. Strengthens the waist, hips, lower back, and thighs.

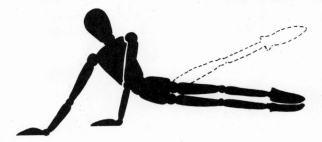

Leg Lifts

Lie on your side with upper body raised and supported by both hands on the floor. Then, keeping upper body and arms straight, raise the top leg straight up and swing it behind your body, then in front of your body.

Return to starting position. Next, roll over on your buttocks to your other side and repeat the movement with the upper leg. Repeat as often as comfortable at a steady pace. You can do a number of leg lifts on one side, then switch to the other side, or alternate sides each time. Strengthens hips, lower back, and thighs.

An alternative exercise from the same position is to hold the top leg high, then lift the bottom leg to meet it. Return to starting position. Alternate sides.

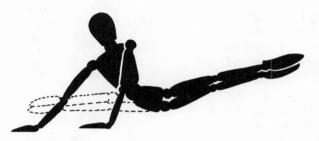

Double Leg Swings

Lie on your side with upper body raised and supported by both hands on the floor. Then, holding legs together, raise them slightly off the floor and swing them all the way around to the other side. You will have to lift your arms momentarily to allow the legs to pass. Repeat as often as comfortable at a steady pace. Strengthens hips, lower back, and thighs.

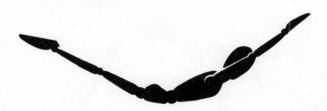

The Swan

Lie face down on the floor with arms and legs fully extended. Then lift your chest, arms, and legs off the floor as high as you can and hold in the up position for a few moments. Return to starting position. Repeat as often as comfortable at a steady pace. Strengthens hips, lower back, and thighs.

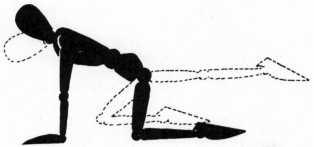

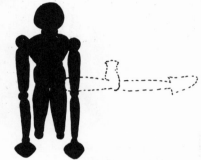

Kneeling Leg Lifts

Get on hands and knees. Then extend one leg to the side, touch toe to the floor, and raise leg as high as you can. Repeat with other leg. Next, extend one leg to the rear (as shown), bend the knee, and raise it as high as possible. Repeat with other leg. Next, extend one leg to the front, lift it as high as possible, then bend the knee and bring it to your chest; now drop your head to meet the knee. Repeat with other leg. Do each phase separately or in sequence as long as comfortable at a steady pace. Strengthens hips, lower back, and thighs.

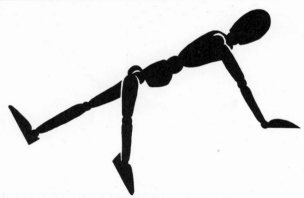

Leg Crossovers (Advanced Exercise)

Lie on your back with body fully extended. Raise body off the floor supported by your heels and hands and arms. Then, keeping legs straight and body raised, cross one leg over the other and touch the toe to one side as far as possible. (You should turn your body with the crossover.) Return to starting position. Repeat with other leg. Repeat sequence as often as comfortable at a steady pace. Strengthens hips, lower back, and thighs.

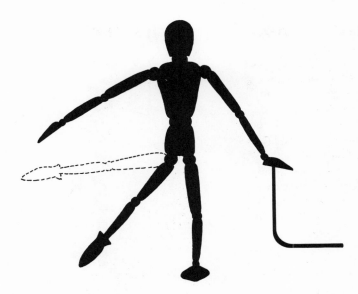

Standing Leg Lifts

Stand with one hand on the back of a chair, a railing, or other such object. Keep your weight on the leg next to the chair, the knee slightly bent. The opposite leg is slightly behind and to the side of your body, held straight with toes only resting easily on the floor. Lift the outside leg as high as you can, then lower it to the floor. Repeat at a steady pace. Next, lift the outside leg to the rear as high as you can, then lower it to the floor. Repeat at a steady pace. Next, lift the outside leg to the front as high as you can, then lower it to the floor. Repeat at a steady pace. Keep your body straight at all times, with head high. Repeat all of these exercises with the opposite leg. Strengthens hips, lower back, and thighs.

Shoulder Stretch

Stand and clasp your hands behind your back as shown. Then raise your arms as high as you can without leaning forward. Hold at highest stretch for a few moments. Relax. Do 3–6 times. Next, bend forward at the waist and bring clasped hands over your head. Hold at full stretch for a few moments. Relax. Do 3–6 times. Stretches shoulder muscles.

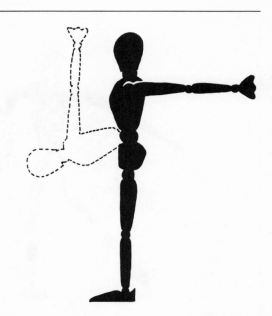

Ankle Stretch

Stand with your body weight resting on one foot. Roll the opposite foot forward and over so it is up on the back of the toes. Then slowly apply your weight to the top of that foot. Relax. Do 2–4 times. Repeat with opposite foot. Stretches the ankles.

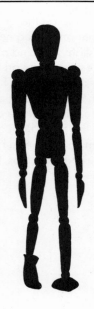

Stand 'n' Stretch

Stand with feet slightly apart, knees bent, and your hands on the floor in front of your toes. Then try to straighten your legs while you keep your hands on the floor. Hold position as long as you can. Next, stand with knees bent and grasp your ankles behind the heels, keeping elbows behind the heels. Then straighten legs while retaining hold on ankles and try to touch your nose to your knees. Hold at maximum stretch for several seconds. Do each exercise 2–4 times. Stretches hip muscles.

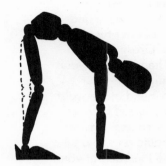

Wide-Straddle Stretch

Sit on the floor with your legs apart, upper body tilted forward, and toes pointed forward. (How far you separate your legs depends on your flexibility. If the knees bend during the pulling and stretching, the legs are too far apart. As you gain flexibility, you will be able to separate your legs farther.) Grasp each ankle with its corresponding hand and

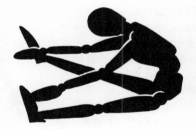

gently pull your body forward as far as you can. Next, grasp one leg with both hands as far down the leg as possible and pull your body as far forward as you can. Repeat grasping other leg. Next, do all three exercises with toes pointing straight up. Hold each stretch for a few moments. Do each stretch 3–5 times. Stretches the back and leg muscles.

Yoga Stretch
(Advanced Exercise)

Sit on the floor with your knees bent outward and the soles of your feet together. Grasp feet with hands. Then, keeping your back straight and your head up, bend at the waist and pull yourself forward. In full stretch position your knees should remain on the floor with the heels of your feet touching your crotch. And when pulling forward, keep your chin up and neck stretched. Do 3–5 times. Stretches hip and back muscles.

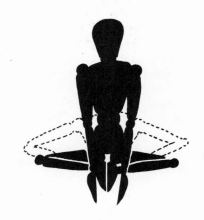

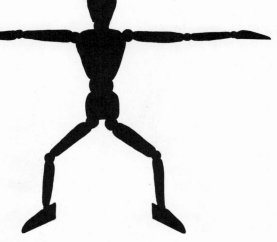

The Elevator

Assume position as shown: knees bent, feet angled outward, arms extended to sides at shoulder level, back straight, head erect. Then lower and raise your body, keeping your knees bent at all times. In lowering, buttocks must not drop below your knees. And knees must remain directly over your feet at all times. Also keep arms extended at all times, and feet and knees at the same angle (as shown). Raise and lower as often as comfortable at a steady pace. Strengthens hips, lower back, and thighs.

Seated Stretch

Sit on the floor with legs together and straight out in front of you. Keeping your back straight, tilt forward at the hips and grasp your ankles, one in each hand. Angle the feet so the toes are pointing forward. Then pull your body forward with your arms and try to touch your navel to your thighs. Hold the stretched position for a few moments. Return to starting position. Do 3–8 times. Stretches the back and hip muscles.

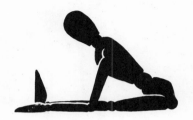

For variety, do the exercise with feet flexed so that toes are pointing straight up.

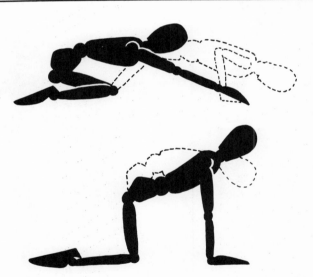

The Cat

Take a kneeling position on the floor with your knees parted and your weight supported by your heels. Stretch your arms forward on the floor as far as you can. Then thrust your body forward, keeping your chin close to the floor. Support your body above the floor on your hands and straighten your elbows and arch your back. Hold the arched position, with abdominal muscles tight, for 3 seconds. Return to the starting position. Do entire sequence 3–7 times. Stretches and strengthens the muscles of the trunk, legs, and arms.

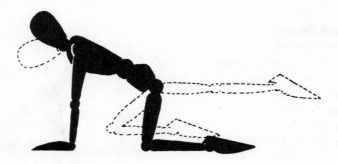

Knee-to-Nose and Kick-Back

Begin on your hands and knees. Drop your head down and bring your right knee up as close to your nose as possible. Then slowly raise your head and at the same time stretch your right leg out behind you as far and as high as you can. Do 4 or more times. Repeat with the left leg. Stretches your back and tightens and firms the buttocks.

The "Rockette"

Stand with your hands on your hips. Then extend your right arm straight out at shoulder level and raise your left leg in front of you with the toes pointed up and touch the fingers of the right hand. Your trunk and pelvis will rotate during the kicking movement. Do 4 times. Repeat with the left arm and right leg. Slims your waistline and tones leg muscles.

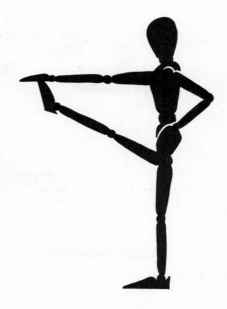

Chest and Shoulder Stretch

Stand with feet about 18 inches apart. Hold a stick, a light rod, a rolling pin, or a rolled-up towel at the ends and behind your back. Then bend forward at the waist, keeping your back straight and your head up. With your hands parallel to each other, pull them upward behind you as high as you can. Relax. Do 5–8 times. Strengthens and stretches the chest, back, and shoulders.

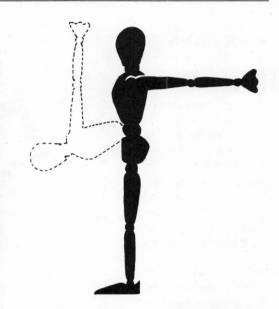

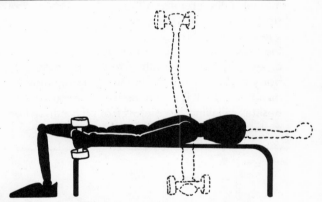

Chest Development

Lie on your back, preferably on a low narrow table or bench, with your feet on the floor. Hold a weight in each hand (a 1-pound dumbbell or a book will do). (The weights offer a degree of resistance to enhance the exercise.) Begin with your hands at your sides. Then: (1) Keeping your arms extended, raise them vertically in front of you and lower them slowly to starting position. (2) Bring arms to vertical position in front of you, then slowly extend them out to the sides at shoulder level. Lower them as far as you can at this point, then return to starting position. (3) Bring arms to vertical position in front of you, then slowly extend them fully above your head. Lower them as far as you can beyond horizontal, then return to starting position. By letting the arms go beyond horizontal in (2) and (3) you get more stretch. Do each of the three parts of the exercise 5–10 or more times, either one at a time or in a 1-2-3 sequence. Strengthens the anterior chest and shoulder girdle muscles.

Pelvic Stretch

Stand the distance of a bent elbow from a wall, with your feet together. Place forearm and palm against the wall at shoulder height. Set the heel of the other hand in the hollow of the buttock. Then contract your abdominal and buttocks muscles strongly while tilting your pelvis backward. Slowly push your hips forward and diagonally toward the wall. Resist the push with the hand on the wall. Hold the final position for a few moments, then return to starting position. Keep your knees straight throughout 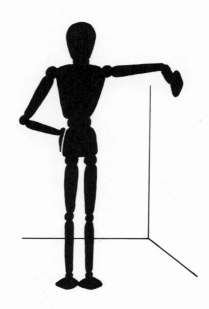 the exercise and your elbow against the wall. When you are pushing hips diagonally forward to the greatest possible extension, avoid twisting your body and touching it to the wall. Do the movement 3 times. Repeat on opposite side. It is recommended the exercise be done 3 times a day. Besides relieving discomfort from dysmenorrhea, the exercise increases mobility of hip joint and stretches hip muscles.

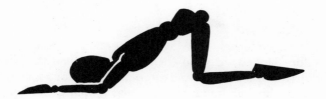

Lower Chest

Kneel on the floor on hands and knees, then bend forward at the hips, with lower arms and hands flat on the floor. Your chest should be touching the floor. Hold this position for as long as comfortable. Do once or twice a day. Helps relieve discomfort of dysmenorrhea.

You might also turn your head from side to side while holding the exercise position.

Abdominal Pump/Pelvic Lift

Lie on your back with knees raised, heels an inch apart. Then, with knees kept together, contract your abdominal and buttocks muscles, rotate your pelvis upward, and raise your hips from the floor. Now distend your abdomen and retract it. Then lower your hips slowly to the starting position. Do 3–6 times. Helps correct a forward pelvic tilt and tones up the abdominal muscles. Also helps relieve discomfort of dysmenorrhea.

For variation, and more relaxation, hold your feet a little apart but keep your knees touching.

11

Machine-Age Exercises

Karen is six months from reaching the big four-oh—the age of forty. And she's worried. Her family is strong, and she's proud of that. Her real estate career is solid, and she enjoys the respect she gets from her peers. But she senses that her body is beginning to show the wear and tear of forty years of life. And she's worried that her energy level isn't what it used to be.

She has increased the frequency of her visits to the Y. She has made a commitment to toning those muscles. Others go to scheduled exercise classes, but Karen finds that impossible. She feels the Nautilus equipment really works for her. She can go any time of the day or evening and do her own routine. She records her activity and progress on cards kept for her at the Y. She is making progress and finds the log a helpful discipline and reinforcement.

Until the mid-1950s, training to enhance muscular strength and endurance was done almost exclusively by lifting "free" weight— barbells and dumbbells. Then there appeared exercise machines based on the principle of variable resistance, whereby the *same degree of muscular effort* when moving weight is maintained *through the entire range of physical motion*. This produces a far more thorough training effect than traditional weight lifting, by virtue of a simple truth of human physics.

When anyone attempts to lift a heavy object—such as a 100-pound barbell—off the floor and above the head, the hardest part of the job is raising it off the floor in the first place and then getting it halfway up. Taking the weight from this point the rest of way requires much less effort, because the arms are now bent and there is much greater, or better, leverage for doing this work. Most of you have experienced this phenomenon in one way or another.

In terms of physical fitness training, the first half of the lift gives a very good workout. The last half gives much less; muscular effort is reduced by about 70 percent. This is where the variable resistance principle comes in. The exercise machines are so designed that the last half of the weight lift (or movement) takes as much effort as the first half. This, of course, affords optimum muscular training.

The exercise machines quickly gained popularity and have become the most widely used form of weight training by recreational physical fitness enthusiasts and professional athletes. Indeed, most YMCAs have separate areas set aside for the machines and have been continuously adding more people to their staffs who are trained specifically to counsel in machine exercise.

The machines have caught on so well not only because they provide more efficient conditioning exercise than traditional weight lifting but also because they are much safer to use. The machines generally have weight stacks that are easily adjustable. The amount of weight you want to move is arranged by merely inserting a pin at the appropriate place in the stack, or otherwise making an uncomplicated adjustment; there is none of the laborious and rather clumsy business of adding or removing heavy iron disks on a weight-lift bar. In this respect the machines are also less time-consuming. And of course, with the machines there is no danger of dropping the weight on a foot.

Furthermore, the operation of the machines themselves is much simpler than with "free" weights, which demand special knowledge and techniques in the way of gripping the bar, setting the feet, and aligning the body. A rank beginner can operate an exercise machine properly the very first time around; they are, in a sense, automatic. This is not to suggest a novice should jump right onto an exercise machine and have a go at it without any qualified instruction on its use. Quite the contrary. There are a number of important considerations for the use of the machines that everyone must be aware of, and we will outline them in a moment.

Because the exercise machines put the muscles through their full range of motion for eight to twelve repetitions, they help you develop strength and endurance without building the "Mr. Universe" musculature associated with traditional "free" weight lifting. This factor, along with safety and ease of operation, has made weight training accessible to a much wider range of people than it has ever been before, and especially to women. Machine exercise can be used for the often exaggerated shaping of muscles mistakenly referred to as "body building" but which has more of a "show biz" character. The machines are essentially for increasing muscular strength and endurance. We should add here that *they are not going to help you lose weight.* If anything, because the machines can help you build up muscle, which is heavier than fat, you could even gain in total body weight. They will, however, help you tone your body for an overall *look* of trimness. And, remember, muscle tissue burns more calories than fatty tissue does.

The exercise machines are manufactured from patented designs. Two of the best known are the Universal Gym Machine and the Nautilus Equipment, although a number of new lines have been introduced in recent years. A Universal machine or any piece of Nautilus equipment can be purchased by an individual, but the cost is fairly prohibitive, which is why such equipment is usually found only in large organizations such as YMCAs. However, a number of other brands of exercise machines are on the market at a more accommodating price. The YMCA is not in a position to evaluate whether these less expensive machines are as sturdy or sophisticated as the Universal or Nautilus equipment.

In any case, most of the machines, including the Universal equipment, function through a system of pulleys and levers. Nautilus, on the other hand, moves the weight stacks (raises and lowers them) via a cam action. Basically, a cam rotates, whereas a pulley and lever system works up and down or back and forth in the process of lifting and lowering weight. Some of the latest machines include the use of a "shock absorber" type of cylinder instead of counterweights. We needn't go any further into the technical aspects of these mechanical differences. The important thing is that in terms of their use for physical conditioning, they all apply the variable resistance principle. However, within this framework there are two opposing views toward weight training with machines, and the YMCA thinks it a good idea that they be discussed here.

Basically, weight training involves working the muscles against resistance. There are two kinds of resistance—positive and negative. Positive is the lifting or pushing of weight; negative is the lowering or releasing of it. A leading proponent of positive resistance, and an advocate of the Universal system he believes is more conducive to it, is Chuck Coker. A onetime U.S. decathlon team member, and coach of twenty-three Olympic medalists, Coker argues that a quick burst of muscular activity in *initiating the movement* of weight—what he calls "ballistics acceleration"—is the most valuable training for muscles involved in the work. He claims that "it requires only $1/10$ of the oxygen to lower a weight than it does to raise (or push) it" and that "only $1/13$ of the bio-chemical activity needed for positive work is required during negative resistance." Therefore, according to Coker, positive resistance builds stronger and more durable muscles.

Arthur Jones, founder of the Nautilus company (the name is taken from the chambered nautilus, a sea mollusk with a shape similar to the cam that is the key to Jones's machines), believes negative resistance is better muscle training. For example, if you are handed a heavy trunk to take down from the tailgate of a truck, you must exert substantial muscular effort to keep the trunk from falling to the ground. Because gravity and downward inertia have rendered the trunk heavier than it would be lifting it up, the effort to keep it from falling gives your muscles the most extensive workout possible. This is the key idea behind negative-resistance training. Accordingly, the emphasis in Nautilus training is the *release* of weight, which has been more or less eased up or out.

In our opinion both positive- and negative-resistance training are, for the most part, of equal value. Indeed, you can obtain either type of resistance on a pulley and lever, cam-action, or shock-absorber machine; it is just a question of emphasis in *initiating* the weight movement, and also perhaps one of personal attitude or taste in training style.

Only in regard to the use of an exercise machine as a rehabilitation tool does the YMCA think there is a significant difference in the kind of machine to use. If you have suffered an injury to a joint or muscle, we think the Nautilus system is better for bringing the body part back to good health. This is because it is a more controlled system. The construction of Nautilus machines is such that in operating them the limbs are in a fixed position. For example, on the wrist-and-forearm machine the elbows must rest firmly on a heavy pad. With Universal machines this element of control is not usually available, and it is necessary to have a therapist with you when using them for body rehabilitation.

In respect to training style, positive resistance tends to be the more aggressive approach. This is reflected not only in the "burst of energy" technique for initiating weight movement, but in the basic exercise pattern. The Universal guidebook specifies that each exercise be repeated ten to fifteen times, in some cases up to twenty times, with little or no pause in between times. What's more, the complete cycle of exercises is to be performed three times at every workout session.

By contrast, in negative-resistance training there is a more relaxed air. The work is done at a slower, more rhythmic pace, and Nautilus training personnel instruct you to initiate the weight movement and release the weight with a gradual, deliberate action. Furthermore, no Nautilus exercise is to be repeated more than twelve times, and the complete cycle is to be performed only once per workout session. These factors may also contribute to the value of Nautilus as a body rehabilitation tool.

YMCA General Recommendations for Exercise on Machines

The YMCA wants to delineate certain procedures and make recommendations for weight training on machines that apply no matter what method you may use—positive or negative resistance or a mix of each.

• It is absolutely essential that when you first take up a machine exercise program you get a full explanation of the system from an expert. It is especially important that you do not begin with too heavy a weight stack. The training counselor is the person to advise you on the amount of weight you should begin with and at what increments you should increase the load. Generally, you begin with the lowest weight load, 10 pounds, and add 5 or 10 pounds to the stack every time you move up as you increase your strength and endurance and your flexibility.

However, a counselor is not going to be with you every time you work out, and of course he or she cannot know at any time how your body actually feels during and after a training session. Thus, you must learn to monitor yourself. The YMCA offers a couple of tips in this respect. The first and second workouts with an increased weight load usually bring some light muscle soreness. This is to be expected, and it will eventually go away as you continue working with that weight load. However, if you feel sharp, intense pain right after a workout, and for a day or so afterward, then you have moved too much weight; you have overdone it and must lighten the load. In any case, it is always safer to use a lighter weight stack and do more repetitions (up to the limit the particular system designates), as there will be less chance of muscle strains and pulls. Not as much force is exerted by this method, which builds more endurance and longer, sleeker muscles. Using a greater weight load and fewer repetitions builds more compact, bunched musculature and greater muscle strength.

• Before beginning any workout session, do a series of warmup exercises, such as stretching or stationary bicycle pumping (if available). Use any of the warmup exercises we have presented in the chapter on calisthenics.

• Do not work on the machines more than three times a week and always take a day off between these sessions. Muscles are well taxed during a good weight-training session, and they must be allowed to rest and recuperate. However, on days off from the machines (or even on days when you have worked on them) you may certainly participate in other physical activity, such as jogging, tennis, basketball, and even calisthenics, although these should emphasize stretching.

• Begin each session by exercising the big-muscle groups—legs, chest, back, shoulders—and conclude with exercises for the small-muscle group—arms, wrists, abdominals, neck.

• The YMCA feels that exercise machines do not provide a truly significant cardiovascular training effect. Advocates of the Nautilus system state that by moving quickly from one machine to the next, some aerobic-type training is achieved. Proponents of the Universal system make an even stronger claim in this regard. They point to the fact that the repetitions are meant to be done one right after the other with hardly a pause in between and that there is little rest in between the different exercises; thus, the heart is given a good workout.

While there may be some aerobic training value in this method or pattern, the YMCA believes it is not enough to offset the potential risk of serious injury. It can be dangerous, especially for beginners, to move weight without sufficient rest periods between repetitions and/or different exercises. The YMCA believes you should do weight training at a comfortable pace and get your aerobic training by the most conventional—and effective—means: jogging, brisk walking, cycling, rope-jumping.

• There are specific exercises that can be done on the machines to train you for particular sports. If your game is golf, tennis, basketball, football, or whatever, inform the training counselor and he will set you up in a routine that will prepare your muscles for the needs of that game.

• Keep in mind that machine exercises are designed primarily for developing muscular strength and endurance. They are not for creating highly pronounced muscle mass, which, in any case, is only for persons with inherently large musculature. A person six feet tall and weighing 145 who is naturally endowed with slender musculature is not going to look like a "Mr. Universe" no matter how much he lifts "free" weight. However, strength and endurance can be achieved by anyone with any body type.

Universal Exercise on Station I—Leg Press (3–5)

This exercises the thigh and knee extensors, hip flexors, and buttocks.

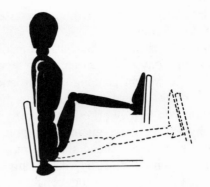

Universal Exercise on Station II—Chest Press (8–12)

This exercises the chest, shoulders, arms, back, abdominals, hips, legs, and buttocks.

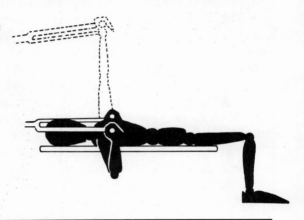

Universal Exercise for Station III—

Shoulder Press (4–6) This exercises the shoulders, arms, legs, and back.

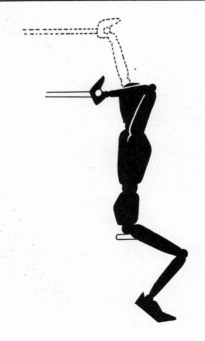

Universal Exercise for Station IV—High Lat (5–8)

This exercises the back, shoulders, arms, and chest.

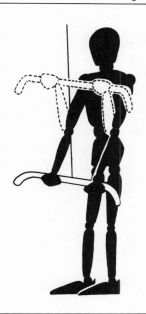

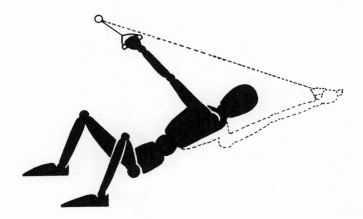

Universal Exercise for Station V—Low Pulley (6–10)

This exercises the shoulders, back, arms, and abdominals.

**Universal Exercise
for Station VI—**
Chinning (3–6)
This exercises the back,
arms, shoulders, and
abdominals.

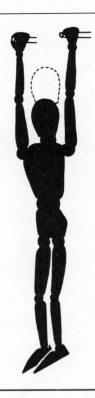

**Universal Exercise
for Station VII—**
Dipping (2–6)
This exercises the back,
shoulders, and upper arms.

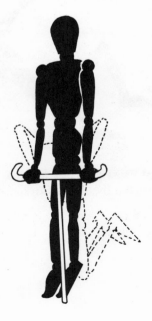

Universal Exercise for Station VIII—Hip Flexor (4–6)

This exercises the hips and abdominals.

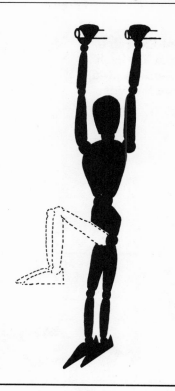

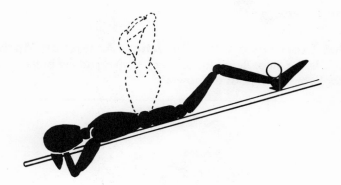

Universal Exercise for Station IX—Abdominal Board (4–10)

This exercises the abdominals and back.

**Universal Exercise
for Station X**—Thigh
and Knee Machine (3–6)
This exercises the thighs.

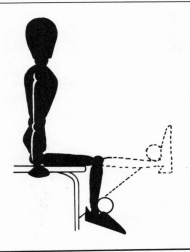

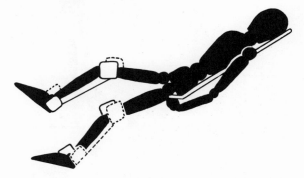

Nautilus Exercises on the Abduction/Adduction Machine
This exercises the inner thighs (adductors). To exercise the outer hips
(abduction), rotate the pads as shown.

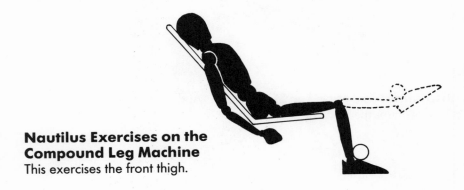

**Nautilus Exercises on the
Compound Leg Machine**
This exercises the front thigh.

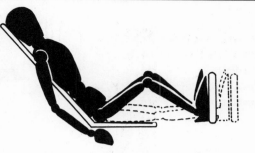

Nautilus Exercise for the Rear Thigh

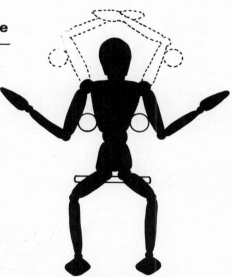

Nautilus Exercise for the Upper and Lower Back—
Arm Machine
This exercises the back and shoulder muscles.

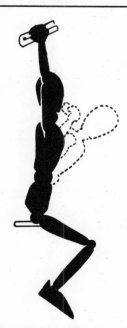

Nautilus Exercise for the Neck, Arms, and Shoulders

Nautilus Exercises on the Double Shoulder Machine

This exercises the shoulder muscles and inner arms.

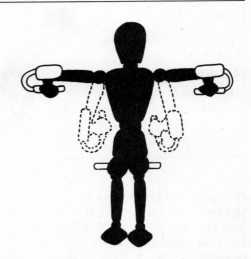

Nautilus Exercise for the Shoulders and Arms

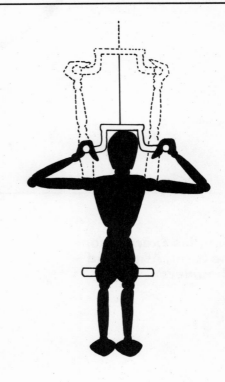

Nautilus Exercise on Rowing—Torso Machine

This exercises the shoulders and back.

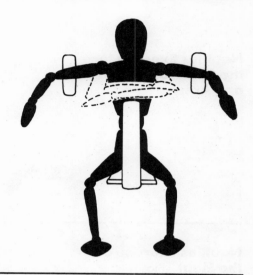

Nautilus Exercises on the Double Chest Machine

This exercises the chest and shoulders.

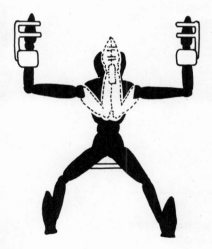

Nautilus Exercise for the Chest, Shoulders, and Arms

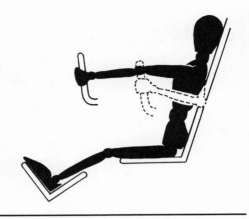

Nautilus Exercise on the Multi—Biceps
Machine
This exercises the arms (front).

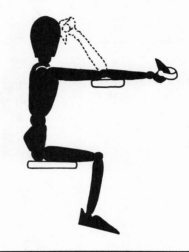

Nautilus Exercise on the Multi—Triceps
Machine
This exercises the arms (rear).

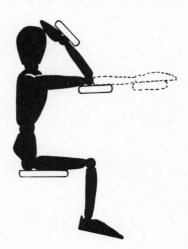

Nautilus Exercise on the Abdominal Machine

This exercises the stomach.

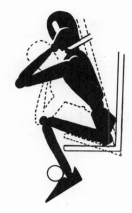

Nautilus Exercise on the Lower Back Machine

This exercises the lower back.

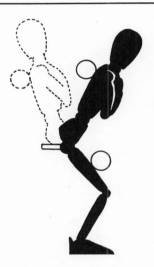

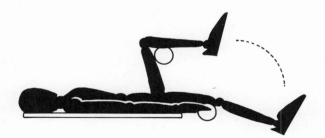

Nautilus Exercise on the Hip and Back Machine

This exercises the legs, hips, and buttocks.

12

Beyond Calisthenics—Sports and Games

One of the exciting things for elementary-school children who play basketball at the Y is to watch the adult league. There is always one retired star who belongs to the Y, and every now and then the kids get a chance to shoot baskets with him.

To the kids, the impressive thing about the pro is where he played and how great he was. The motivator for adults is how the pro has stayed in shape and how well he still plays!

It is generally agreed that a person cannot achieve a high level of physical fitness *only* playing games or doing athletic activities, that one cannot play oneself into all-around good shape. Swimming may come the closest to providing a complete physical workout, but just about every other sport will miss a few major muscle groups, and many provide only minimal cardiovascular/aerobic training. It is for this reason that physical fitness experts will counsel that a person who wants to get into better condition should begin with conventional exercises. This is sound advice, but not the final word.

It is quite possible that by beginning your fitness odyssey with participation in a sport you will be inspired to add on the "gym" work of push-ups, chin-ups, stretching, and strength and endurance exercises. It is the nature of most of us to want to perform well, or better, at sports, and it doesn't take very long on a basketball or tennis court, on a track or a ski slope, to realize that you will be more adept and more competitive if you develop more flexibility, more muscular strength, and a stronger heart than the sport itself can give you. Needless to say, the wise athlete gets into exercising as a way to prevent injuries on the playing field.

There are no statistics on the subject, but our guess is that a great many of the people now part of the explosion of interest in exercise entered into it *after* having taken up jogging or running, skiing, tennis, or racquetball. Sports are a kind of sugar-coated way to get into a physical fitness program. You know a sport is going to be more interesting, exciting, and intellectually stimulating than calisthenics or weight-lifting. Some of that enthusiasm may be rooted in nonathletic superficialities—a desire to expand one's social life with tennis parties or weekend skiing trips, or to buy some new and perhaps trendy clothes. Then again, taking up a sport gives one an opportunity to be a kid again. Many find that their playing days did not end, after all, when they left school. What's more, with physical and emotional maturity, they turn out to be better players than they were when young.

There is yet another aspect to sports that is more subtle, but is perhaps the most meaningful of all. In his famous book *Homo Ludens* [Man the Player]: *A Study of the Play Element in Culture,* Dutch social historian Johan Huizinga pointed out some virtues of play. For example, play tends to be beautiful, with a rhythm and harmony of movement. Also, there is a ritual in playing games that is concomitant with a demand for order. Games are played by a clear set of rules that everyone must accept or there is no game. Games, then, appeal to our aesthetic sense and our need for a degree of control which we may not always derive from our work or personal relationships, where the rules are never quite as precise.

Huizinga wrote: "Play is a thing by itself. The play-concept as such is of a higher order than seriousness. For seriousness seeks to exclude play, whereas play can very well include seriousness."

From playing games we may experience tension, the need for poise, balance, control, solution, and resolution (a clear-cut beginning, middle, and end), yet in a forgiving context, for we know too that it does not mean anything. When the game is over, it is over, and we go on with life. But we have had a valuable release and expression of intrinsic human drives.

If any or all of the above moves us, consciously or subconsciously, to play games, it is not a bad thing. And if playing games leads us to a full-scale fitness program, a very good thing has happened.

You may be predisposed in your choice of an athletic activity by past experience, physical capabilities, a taste for something slow or fast.

Whatever the reason, the sport or sports you choose may not give as much physical training as others. But you will get some. Even golf, a popular game for people over thirty but one of the least exertive, requires three times the energy used for sitting in a chair (assuming you walk your eighteen holes). And you will burn a few more calories if you hit practice balls a couple of hours a week.

In any event, there are definite differences in how much overall energy is consumed and how many muscle groups are exercised by various games and athletics. We are going to outline those and other factors for a number of activities usually taken up by recreational athletes in their postschool years.

In all sports activity, though, we want to emphasize that the conditioning value is not entirely dependent on how well you play a game. In tennis, for example, the ability of the other player is a factor in the quality of the workout, but on the whole an "all-American" does not get a better workout than an average player. The key is in how often and for how long you play. You will find in Appendices 1 and 2 some tables showing the overall and the specific conditioning values of a number of games/athletics.

With weight control in mind, as well as cardiovascular training, Appendices 1 and 3 show how many calories each athletic activity consumes. Be advised that the computations are not absolute. There are many variables that make it impossible to render a precise number of calories expended for any activity. For example, if you swim in very cold water, the caloric cost increases because you need energy to maintain body temperature. And how fast you jog or run—the intensity of your performance—will determine the number of calories you use. Still, the figures we present are reasonably close to a median and can serve as a guide.

Furthermore, in respect to the calorie-consumption figures, keep in mind the amount of calories you need daily. The simplest way to compute your need is to multiply your total body weight by 15. Thus, a 170-pound man who is moderately active will need 2,550 calories a day *to maintain his present weight.* If activity increases, so does the caloric requirement, *and vice versa.* However, young people need more calories in proportion to their size. For example, boys from fourteen to eighteen years old who weigh 130 and are 5'5" tall need 3,000 calories a day; girls sixteen to eighteen at 119 pounds and 5'2" need 2,300 calories daily.

We will also include in this chapter nutrition tips and reminders directed especially to athletes.

In-the-Water Sports

SWIMMING

There is virtually universal agreement that swimming is just about the best athletic activity in terms of physical conditioning. It is excellent for developing cardiovascular fitness because of the work involved against the resistance of the water. Studies have shown that heart size increases when a person swims for any length of time, and maximum oxygen uptake is increased accordingly.

The steady and rhythmic movement of the muscles of the upper body develops the strength and flexibility of those muscles, and swimming is an especially good activity for the back. By using some swim-stroke variations of the standard crawl, such as the breaststroke and back-stroke, the lower body and legs are also well exercised. Also, the YMCA has developed a program known as Physical Fitness Through Water Exercise that can be used to strengthen muscles.

Because there is no weight bearing on the joints, swimmers are much less susceptible to the muscle soreness and tightness often experienced by runners and the tennis elbow and strained or torn ligaments that other sports might inflict. The swimming action has a massaging effect on the legs that helps avoid varicose veins.

The cool water is always refreshing, and swimming is the preferred exercise during exceptionally hot weather.

Calories burned when swimming have been estimated as follows:

Breaststroke	7–11	calories per min.
Backstroke	8–11.5	calories per min.
Crawl	9–14	calories per min.

It is advisable to do some warmup exercises before beginning a swimming session. Recommended are jumping jacks, torso and lower leg stretches, and shoulder rolls. It is not a good idea to dive into cold water at the start if your body is quite warm, as the shock of a sudden temperature change might be dangerous. No cool-down is required, though, because the hydrostatic effect of the water prevents blood from pooling in the extremities.

Swimming does have some drawbacks. You need a good-sized pool (competition length is ideal), and even then the lanes must be kept free of frolickers to allow for undisturbed lap swimming.

And of course, you must know how to swim reasonably well, since a bit of paddling about is not going to be of any fitness value. If you are not a strong swimmer, however, you can swim a length of the pool, walk back to the other end, swim another length, and so on, and obtain good exercise. Otherwise, swim in the shallower water of a pool and near the shore of a lake or ocean.

Swimming is a solitary exercise, but this might be another advantage for people who work in a busy environment all day. The aloneness in the water—and just the effect of the water—can be very relaxing for the emotions.

On the whole, swimming causes very few joint problems. However, the overhead swing of the arms during the crawl stroke might bring an irritation of the rotator cuff, which is the joint at which the arm and shoulder meet. This is much more common among baseball pitchers because of the forceful twisting of the throwing arm. Tennis players may also suffer this problem from the serving motion, which is similar to that of a baseball pitcher. Rotator cuff irritation is difficult to lose. The healing process requires total rest for an extensive period of time.

On-the-Water Sports

CANOEING, KAYAKING, ROWING

The mechanics of rowing require that the leg and back muscles be as vigorously involved as the arm and shoulder muscles. And boats equipped with sliding seats increase the use of the trunk of the body.

Canoeing and kayaking mainly involve the arm muscles, the wrists and hands, the shoulders, and the back in a rather limited way.

Of the three, rowing probably provides the best overall exercise in terms of a fitness program, although white-water canoeing can offer some vigorous exertion over a short period of time.

An estimate has been worked up for the number of calories expended while rowing:

51 strokes per min.	4.1 calories per min.
87 strokes per min.	7.0 calories per min.
97 strokes per min.	11.2 calories per min.

Racket Games

TENNIS

To get a sufficient physical workout in tennis, it is important to play with those of equal ability. If the disparity is great enough, the better player will not get nearly the work of the lesser one. Singles tennis generally takes more exertion than doubles.

It is only when the play at tennis (be it singles or doubles) is steady and varied, when there are long rallies or exchanges to decide points and the shots make the players run to reach balls, that tennis provides a significant cardiovascular workout. On the whole, the game is one of short bursts of activity. However, better tennis players will be in almost constant motion even when waiting for an opponent to hit the ball—they do a lot of short-hopping in place—because this helps prepare for movement to the ball when it does come. In doing this the exercise value of the game is increased.

Playing the game itself stretches and strengthens the shoulder and forearm (of the playing side only), the thighs, and the calf muscles. The muscles of the lower back and groin get a good stretch. However, *these very areas are the most susceptible to injury if they are not in good condition before you play,* so it is vital that you do other forms of exercise for them. Special emphasis should be put on working the shoulder of the hitting arm, which is used extensively in the tennis serve. The overhead swing of the arm can cause problems in the rotator cuff. As mentioned earlier, baseball pitchers have the same problem, as their motion is very similar to that of tennis serving.

Perhaps the most chronic physical problem in tennis is injury to the ligaments and tendons around the elbow of the hitting arm, which is known as tennis elbow. There seems to be no exercise to prevent this. The best way to avoid tennis elbow is to try to hit the ball as often as possible in the center of the racket. Off-center hits cause the racket to twist, and the elbow with it; hence the injury. It is also advisable to use either a wooden racket or one made with a graphite frame. Both absorb the shock of mis-hit balls better than a steel-framed racket. (Graphite is rather expensive, but if you play enough, it is worth the investment.)

Calories burned at tennis are estimated as follows:

Singles	7–8 calories per min.
Doubles	5–6 calories per min.

You should definitely do some stretching exercises before taking to the tennis court. Stretch the arms and back, and the hamstrings in particular. A cold start in tennis can cause muscle pulls and tears.

While tennis does not generally give the vigorous overall workout of jogging or swimming, it is a good test of hand-eye coordination and calls for a variety of strokes, well-thought-out strategy, and quick decision-making. It also has a socializing character that reflects the game's origins as one played "in society." We should add, though, that tennis has become quite democratized in the past decade or so. The "snobbish" quality it once had is not as prevalent anymore.

RACQUETBALL

Racquetball has become very popular in the past few years, many of its newer players having come over from tennis, which they found a bit more technically demanding. In comparison to tennis, racquetball is easier to play reasonably well if you have had no previous racket-game experience. Most YMCAs in the North find that racquetball courts are the single most popular sports areas in the winter.

Racquetball is another game of short bursts of intensive energy, but the rest periods are quite brief—it is a fast-paced game—so the overall cardiovascular training is good, probably a little better than tennis. Strength is not a big factor in playing this game, but endurance is, as well as flexibility.

The game calls for frequent rapid changes of direction to hit shots and reach those of your opponent. The steady twisting and turning that this entails, and the fact that the game is played a lot of the time in a semi-crouch, puts heavy strain on the low-back, pelvic, thigh, and calf muscles. It is very important to get all these areas into good condition with various stretching and strength and endurance exercises prior to playing. If not, you stand a good chance of suffering muscle pulls and tears, low-back pain, and torn or severely strained tendons. Tennis elbow is not a great worry, though, because the racquetball stroke is made largely with the wrists and hands, with the hitting arm bent. Moreover, the stroke tends to be a short one, so more balls are hit solidly.

Calories burned at racquetball average between 7 and 13 per minute.

SQUASH

The fact that squash courts are usually assigned for periods of no more than forty-five minutes attests to its vigor; no one needs more time than that to get a complete, exhaustive athletic workout. Squash is the fastest paced of all the racket games and consequently the best for cardiovascular training. By the same token, it puts a proportionately greater stress on the low-back, pelvic, thigh, and calf muscles, and these areas must be conditioned prior to play. In squash the twisting and turning and changes of direction are all the more demanding for their greater frequency. At the same time, squash may be more fun than tennis or racquetball for the very reason that it is so fast and constant.

Squash is a much older game than racquetball—about as old as tennis—and has long been a favorite in Great Britain and at eastern universities in the United States. There has been wider interests in squash in recent years, but it is still relatively unknown by the general public. Like racquetball, squash is played only in an enclosed court (indoors), with the ball played to and off four walls (in racquetball you can also use the ceiling, but not in squash). The squash ball is much smaller in size, and firmer, so shots have considerable velocity. If you are struck by a hard-hit ball, some injury can occur. On the whole, though, squash is not a dangerous game unless you are not in good condition before going on court.

Estimated calories burned at squash are 10 to 12 per minute.

HANDBALL

Technically, handball is not a racket game. It *is,* however, if you consider the hand as a form of racket. In fact, handball is the forerunner of tennis and other racket games, having been played by twelfth-century monks in their monasteries as spring fertility rites. A racket gradually evolved to replace, or extend, the human hand because it made hitting the ball easier. That is probably why handball is not as popular as tennis, racquetball, or squash; it is harder to play.

Handball requires the same physical attributes as the other racket games—strength, agility, flexibility. And because you must move up closer to the ball in order to hit it, handball is a good cardiovascular workout.

In order to prevent injuries, you need the same preconditioning exercises for handball as for the other racket games.

Handball will burn about the same number of calories as squash—10 to 12 per minute.

Ball Games

VOLLEYBALL

Volleyball was originated by YMCA leaders in Holyoke, Massachusetts, in 1895 and was closely associated with the YMCA for many years afterward; it is still part of YMCA athletic programs. Volleyball is a popular game if only because it requires no special or outstanding athletic skills to play it reasonably well, and men seem to have no advantage over women. At the same time, it is a rather mild game as a physical exercise except when played in a highly competitive way. It is especially good for flexibility, but only fair as cardiovascular training, since even in the most competitive games most of the players on each side are not directly participating in the movement of the ball. At best, volleyball is a "short burst of energy" game.

Still, it is a decent enough workout and a lot of fun on the beaches and at camps during the summer months; it does not take up much room, and it requires very little equipment and nothing more than a simple patch of ground for a playing surface.

Estimated calorie expenditure for volleyball ranges from 5–10 calories per minute.

BASKETBALL

Basketball, a game invented at the YMCA college in Springfield, Massachusetts (in 1891), by Dr. James Naismith, a YMCA physical education instructor, is the one *team* sport from which the recreational athlete can expect the most complete fitness workout. It offers an excellent cardiovascular exercise by virtue of the almost continuous running that the game entails. In addition, the jumping, quick stops and starts, and changes of direction enhance flexibility. All these attributes are heightened, or perhaps exaggerated, when the game is played "one on one" or "two on two" in only half a court.

Because it is such a high-intensity game, however, basketball may not be for most persons over forty who have not been physically active right up to the moment. If you are over forty and in top-notch condition, with good oxygen uptake and body flexibility, basketball will serve to keep you in fine shape and will give you a vigorous competitive format.

The main precaution for the game is the maintenance of strength and flexibility in the legs. Knee and ankle injuries are the bane of basketball players' existence.

Otherwise, the game is readily accessible, with many outdoor courts in parks and playgrounds (and hoops over garage doors). Personal equipment needs are minimal and relatively inexpensive—a ball and a pair of gym shoes.

The calorie-burn rate for basketball has a little wider range than nonteam sports. The pace of the game can be influenced by varying personalities among the players and the style and strategy of play. Thus, the estimated calorie consumption rate is between 10 and 13 calories per minute.

The Pedal Sports

WALKING, JOGGING, RUNNING

We said earlier that the prescribed way to begin getting into good physical condition when starting from poor condition is to walk. Walking often leads to jogging, and quite a few joggers move on to running. Whether or not you make the complete transition, the three modes of pedal transportation/exercise are closely related in terms of conditioning and share the fact that, unlike most athletic activities, they do not need preconditioning; the very acts of walking, jogging, and running develop fitness for walking, jogging, and running.

The ultimate objective in walking as exercise is to do two miles in thirty minutes. This will result in an energy expenditure equal to a good calisthenics or jogging workout, although it will take a little longer. For most people this walking pace should induce a heart rate of 120 to 130 beats per minute (bpm). The rate should not be above that, so watch for overstress by regularly taking your pulse. The pulse rate should drop below 120 bpm within three minutes after exertion. If you find you are overstressed, slow down your pace of walking *but always walk the prescribed distance*—two miles, four miles, or whatever you have decided to do.

The YMCA's walking schedule for fitness beginners is to walk three times a week for ten weeks. This schedule is flexible, depending on how your personal fitness develops.

Walking will exercise most muscle groups, although the arms and chest get somewhat less of a workout. This can be raised by swinging your arms vigorously while walking. (In the warmup and cool-down exercises we have described, there are other exercises you can do while walking.)

When walking, be cognizant of the terrain you cover. Uphill is going to require more energy, of course, and even the surface itself will have a bearing—a smooth concrete or asphalt surface will require about three quarters of the energy needed to walk across a plowed field.

Calorie-burn estimates for walking on level ground are:

2	mph	3 calories per min.
3	mph	4.5 calories per min.
3.5	mph	5.5 calories per min.
4	mph	6.5 calories per min.

Jogging is a peculiarly American "invention" and surely one of the most popular physical fitness activities to come along in many years. It knows no age barriers, costs very little money, can be done anywhere at any time in any sort of weather. And except for the very real potential for injury to the legs and feet, jogging is an excellent aerobic exercise and calorie burner. It is a good way to trim your body composition *when accompanied by a proper diet.*

Jogging is really a slower, easier form of running. At what point jogging becomes running is not clear, but Jim Fixx, the well-known running guru, has said that "running is supposed to be a pace faster than eight minutes a mile and jogging any pace that is slower." Most people begin jogging at between 4.5 and 5 mph, which puts it a step ahead of your top walking pace. However, the jogging technique is closer to running than walking. We will assume everyone knows a walk from a jog from a run.

The average jog is for less than an hour a day. Usually a training stimulus is attained when the heart rate goes above 135 bpm.

You should jog with your head up, your body upright, your arms bent and slightly away from your body. If you jog on a banked path, say just inside the curb of a street, on the return you should jog along the same path to prevent stress on one side of the body caused by continually leaning one way. This holds true especially if you jog on a banked indoor track.

Breathe steadily and normally. Dr. Kenneth Cooper has pointed out that the old notion that runners should breathe in through the nose and out through the mouth restricts athletic performance. So does pursed-lip breathing, gasping, and trying to run at a pace where you take a certain number of steps for each breath.

When you feel your jog is complete, stop and begin walking to bring your body back from the stress point. Do not stop cold.

Clothing for jogging should be simple and light. Even in cold weather it is not advisable to wear rubberized or sweat-retaining garments. Remember, true weight is lost by burning calories, not by losing body water. You should definitely wear a hat in cold weather, though, since half the body's heat loss is through the scalp.

Most important of all, though, is that you have a good pair of shoes for jogging (and running). The sole should have plenty of cushion, since most people jog on hard surfaces. A rippled sole is preferable, according to Dr. Cooper. Tennis sneakers are not recommended because they are constructed with rounded edges to facilitate side-to-side movement, and since joggers only run forward, they need shoes with more rigid side support. Be sure the shoe is wide enough and long enough to accommodate the movement of the foot during the activity—a shoe too tight will cause problems—and make sure it has a good arch support, especially if you have flat feet. Knee aches are often the result of shoes with poor arch supports. Finally, the shoe should fit snugly around the heel, which might be raised slightly. There are many brands of shoes on the market that are constructed specifically for jogging/running, so finding a good pair should not be difficult.

Wearing the proper shoes and jogging whenever possible on softer surfaces will help prevent the injuries common to jogging—injuries that are exacerbated by running. We will discuss them shortly in the section on running.

In the meantime, don't let the worry of injury stop you from jogging. It is excellent exercise, and not as solitary as you might think. Many joggers jog together. There are those who say that if you can hold a conversation with a mate, you are jogging; if you can't, you are running.

The calorie-burn estimate for jogging is 9 calories per minute at 5 mph.

The surge in running interest is indicated by the increased number of marathon races being staged and the huge numbers of entrants in each. This may be seen as reflecting our competitive nature and a detraction from the fitness aims of the activity, but our observation is that most recreational runners who enter the marathons do not expect to win. They seem to get pleasure out of the ambience, and simply being able to go the distance is victory enough.

When we speak of running here, we have in mind distance, or endurance, running, which is a fitness activity as compared to shorter runs or dashes, which are strictly for competition. The problems associated with running are the physical injuries that can develop from it. In *Sports for Life* Drs. Robert Buxbaum and Lyle Micheli write: "Running has been the main sport responsible for the rapid expansion of sports medicine programs. Most of the specialists in this area [are] orthopedists . . . and podiatrists . . . [whose] clinics are full of people whose feet, knees, hips, shins and other lower extremity parts are aching, tight, swollen, or bruised."

These patients are runners. They suffer blisters from poorly fitted shoes, and "runners' toes"—hemorrhages under the toenails caused by the repeated trauma of jamming the toes against the front of their shoes. If you run, be sure your toenails are clipped and your shoes fit properly.

Shin splint is another common occurrence among runners. A shin splint may be a stress fracture, a small crack in the tibia. Do not run if you feel sharp pain there. Rest to let it heal.

Hip injuries are not uncommon, especially among people who have unequal leg lengths, which itself is fairly common. This can be corrected by putting a lift in the shoe for the shorter leg.

Back problems are also a worry for runners—muscle spasms, irritation of the sciatic nerve or a low-back disk. The jarring of impact while running may not cause these problems but will bring them forward more readily.

All the above makes it seem as though running is a very dangerous activity. It is not, so long as you wear proper footgear and ease slowly into the activity by walking, then jogging, and then running at relaxed paces.

The estimated calorie-burn for running is as follows:

5.5 mph   10.5 calories per min.
7   mph   12.5 calories per min.

SKIING (DOWNHILL AND CROSS-COUNTRY)

Skiing downhill was a better conditioning activity when it was first being done in the United States, around the turn of the century. At that time, skiers had to make their way on foot to the top of the slope. The great growth in skiing interest since then is surely due in large part to the development of mechanical lifts that carry skiers up the hill or mountain. But, ironically, what is good for the skiing business detracts from the sports fitness value.

Caloric expenditure for a ski run is high. It would take around 600 calories per hour, but only if the run lasted that long. It usually goes for about five minutes, making it an interrupted activity that is not the cardiovascular workout of jogging, running, or cross-country skiing. Nonetheless, the physical demands of downhill skiing are impressive. One needs a flexible body and much muscular strength throughout to maintain body position and control during a descent and to muster the brief power bursts needed to make turns and negotiate "moguls" (hillocks of snow resulting from the carving action of skis on steep slopes).

You must bring those physical attributes with you to the slopes, though. The skiing itself will help condition the legs and arms, but otherwise the activity uses more than it creates in terms of physical conditioning. Indeed, if you are not fit, there is a high risk of injury from falls that come with fatigue. Skiers begin their training for a season well in advance with running or jogging, rope-jumping, wall-sitting, and other flexibility and strength and endurance exercises. Many YMCAs offer an excellent program titled Get Fit to Ski. It is also important to do warmup exercises at the ski site.

Studies have shown that the fitness of the skier and the setting and condition of the ski bindings are the two keys to preventing injury. It is of utmost importance that you have a ski-to-boot binding system whereby the skis will release readily when a fall occurs. Many serious injuries occur when a skier falls and his skis remain attached to his feet.

It should go without saying that any first attempts at skiing must be preceded by instruction and practice at the sport. In a sense, trying to stand upright and move about on a slippery surface wearing slats of wood as long as your body is a somewhat unnatural act. What's more, with some skill going for you, you will be more relaxed emotionally at the start of a run; anxiety causes skiing spills just as readily as does poor physical condition or an error.

Skiing is dependent on plenty of good snow, and snow-making machines can provide what nature doesn't. And the equipment for the sport, as well as travel to and staying at the site (which is usually far from home), is generally expensive. But the thrill of zooming over crisp snow down a mountain in scenic country can be exhilarating. And despite all the caveats stated here, it is also good exercise.

The estimated calorie consumption for a downhill ski run is from 6 to 10 calories per minute.

Cross-country, or Nordic, skiing has gained a considerable following in recent years. Perhaps many of the adherents are people who wanted the scenery, the clear winter air, the exercise, but not the cost, travel time, risk of injury, and technical skill that downhill skiing demands. Although cross-country skiing can't match the thrill of a downhill run on skis, it is in every other way a superb alternative. In fact, as an exercise for fitness, cross-country skiing ranks equally with running and swimming and easily outdistances downhill skiing in this respect.

The beauty of the sport is that you don't need mountainous terrain; thus, you can participate on a golf course, in the woods, or in an open field near home. Cost is also reduced by the relatively modest equipment expense and the fact that you don't need to wear as much clothing as downhill skiers do. Cross-country skiing generates a lot of body heat, and participants usually avoid heavy down jackets and leggings, opting instead for clothing that allows perspiration to evaporate; a heavy sweater, a windbreaker, a hat, and mittens usually suffice, along with a knapsack to stow clothing in when the body gets too warm and a sandwich for when it gets hungry.

To ski cross-country style you need only a routine sense of balance, but a good cardiovascular system before you start. Muscular strength is also necessary, but this will be developed by the activity itself. So will an even better cardiovascular function; there have been estimates of up to 1,000 calories an hour expended while skiing cross-country, and oxygen uptake is similar to that of a long-distance runner.

The upper body gets a good muscular workout, especially the shoulders and arms, which manipulate the ski poles to push you forward with steady, continuous strokes.

Injuries are mainly to the legs and hips, but the boots are low and soft compared to the rigid ones downhill skiers use, and since falls are less violent anyway, the activity is reasonably safe.

The estimated average calorie-burn for cross-country skiing is 7.5 to 15 calories per minute.

ICE SKATING/ROLLER SKATING

Skating doesn't require any special cardiovascular preparation, and except for strong ankles and thighs you don't need much muscular strength, endurance, or flexibility; anyone in average good condition can handle skating exercise.

However, you must know how to skate reasonably well, for slow, casual skating does not make for a significant training stimulus. If you have always wanted to skate but never got around to it, or skated when you were young but have gotten away from it, a few lessons and some practice will get you going.

You should do some stretching exercises just before getting on the rink, especially for the lower body.

The injuries in skating come primarily from falls. Improving your skating ability is one antidote to this, but a better one (since even good skaters take a flop now and then) is to *learn how to fall*. If you do it a relaxed way and try to break the force of impact by rolling with the fall, injuries will be much less severe.

Ice skating is a particularly pleasant experience, and it is quite inexpensive when done in the quiet of a frozen stream or pond on a crisp afternoon. It is a moderate exercise that is a worthy diversion in your total fitness program.

The recreational skater going at a fairly fast pace for three or four miles at a time will consume anywhere from 5 to 10 calories a minute.

BICYCLING

Bicycling ranks near the top as an aerobic/cardiovascular sport. Going a mere 6 mph on a level road will burn 300 calories an hour. The steady pumping action also give the legs, hips, lower back, and abdomen excellent exercise, and the bicycling will serve to get your body into good condition. No preconditioning is really necessary, so long as you begin cycling slowly and over short distances if you are just starting your fitness program. Indeed, part of preconditioning involves use of the stationary bicycle, a device that can be used throughout your life.

Pain in the upper back and neck can occur among cyclists who use the racer-style handlebars, which require a lot of head twisting to check on traffic behind. A rear-view mirror solves that difficulty. You don't have to have a racer-type bicycle, and even a tricycle will serve you well. Many senior citizens use "trikes" to get around and keep in shape.

Very few of us have not had the bicycling experience as youths, when it was a splendid means to express our independence with easy and relatively long-range mobility. With our bikes we could explore new places far from home—another part of the big city, the next town down the road. The bicycle made us travelers. It can serve the same purpose for adults, for bicycling permits a slower and more penetrating observation of what we bike through, by, over. And of course, if you learned to cycle as a youth you never forget how.

Using the bicycle as a practical source of transportation to and from work is more in the European than the American tradition, but as the fossil-fuel energy problem develops, we may have more Americans pedaling to and fro. Regardless of why it's done, bicycling gives good exercise at low cost.

Energy consumption for bicycling has been estimated as follows:

6 mph	4.5 calories per min.
8 mph	5.5 calories per min.
10 mph	6.5 calories per min.

HIKING

Hiking, you might say, is walking with a larger purpose. Hikers have a definite destination *away from* where they start out. But the hike is more involved in other ways. It is generally done over uneven terrain—in woods, along the sides or up into mountains and hills. It means carrying camping equipment or at least a knapsack full of food, drink, some basic medical supplies, and matches. By virtue of all these factors, hiking becomes more of a game than simply walking. As an exercise it gives all the benefits that walking does, only more so.

Clothing is an important consideration when hiking. Boots must be sturdy for good ankle support. Their soles should be made of hard rubber and treaded to offer protection against rocks and roots and for going up and down steep hills. The boots must fit well, of course, and when you buy a pair, be sure you are wearing two pairs of socks you will use when hiking—a thin cotton pair underneath a heavier woolen pair to keep moisture away from the feet.

Otherwise, hiking clothes should be sensibly suited to the climate you are hiking in, with sudden changes in temperature and wind conditions fitted into the equation. Hiking in mountain areas can be especially tricky in this regard, and you must always be aware of how high you are—the higher the air, the thinner it is, which affects your cardiovascular capacity.

Energy consumption is quite variable for hiking. The nature of the terrain has much to do with how many calories you will burn, but rest assured you will burn more than a few.

Hiking is for those who want to get close to nature. There is no better way.

DANCING

The traditional view of athletics, held for centuries, has been that the necessary power, speed afoot, agility, and endurance were a "manly" business, even for women, an expression of *machismo* delivered with unvarnished force. While the graceful athlete has always been appreciated and applauded when he wins, it is when the big-boned, brawny player knocks over opponents with sheer—if inelegant—might that the cheers ring through the rafters.

But times are changing. We now hear sports commentators utter what would have been unimaginable only a few years ago, that the *dancer* Rudolf Nureyev may be the greatest *athlete* in the world. What's more, football teams, those bastions of he-manship, are including ballet in their training; they are learning basic movements from classic dance as a way to increase coordination, agility, speed afoot, and at the same time get cardiovascular training for strength and endurance.

Thus, we include dancing as a sport/athletic activity. We refer primarily to what is called Choreographed Exercise, which is not meant to teach people new steps to use in a ballroom, but provides an opportunity to put the body joints through a full range of motion, to exercise arm and leg muscles, the trunk and neck, all to the rhythm of taped or recorded music.

Actually, recreational dancing is also good exercise, as the following table indicates:*

Dance	Calories per Minute
Fox-Trot	5.2
Waltz	5.7
Twist/Disco	6.25
Rhumba	7.0
Charleston	8.06
Polka	9.0

But Choreographed Exercise, which does not require knowing the intricacies or the social arrangements of most recreational dances, provides the greater exercise. The calorie-burn rate is estimated as follows:

	Calories per Minute
Low-Level Dancing	3.96 (women)
	4.17 (men)
Medium-Level Dancing	6.28 (women)
	6.86 (men)
High-Level Dancing	7.75 (women)
	9.48 (men)

You might look into a Choreographed Exercise program. Most local YMCAs offer the program. They're known by many different names, but all are excellent. Basically, they are exercise movements with a dance flavor, accompanied by music.

Nutrition Tips for Athletics/Games-Playing

• "Quick-energy" foods—sweets such as honey or candy bars—eaten just before participation do not enhance performance in short

*Adapted from *The Cardiologists Guide to Fitness & Health*, by Drs. Lenore Zohman, Albert Kattus, and Donald Softness (New York: Simon & Schuster)

duration/low energy-cost athletic events. The sugar will be digested within minutes and, in fact, can leave you depleted nutritionally and emotionally.

• Complex carbohydrates such as starches—in potatoes and pasta, for example—put sugar (glucose) into the system when broken down during digestion. However, the process is much slower than with "sugar foods" and therefore provides long-term energy plus real nutritional value. It is generally recommended that an athlete's diet should consist of 55 to 60 percent carbohydrates.

• Protein *is not* a primary source of muscular energy, and eating a big steak before "the game" is a poor idea. It will take too long to digest, and, among other things, it can cause dehydration.

• When replacing fluids lost through perspiration, drink cool plain water (although such drinks as Gatorade are okay). Do not drink sugary beverages such as colas, or take salt tablets! You might take bouillon or broth to replace lost sodium and liquid while still participating in the activity, but water is best.

• Wait at least two hours after a *heavy* meal before exercising vigorously. It takes that long for the blood to resume normal distribution. You risk heart stress, otherwise. A light meal (mainly fluids) does not take nearly as long to digest.

• "There is no scientific evidence at the present time to indicate that athletic performance can be improved by modifying a basically sound diet." Dr. Herbert deVries, Exercise Physiologist, UCLA.

• Tables describing the fitness potential of various popular sports are found in Appendices 1 and 2. A table giving the approximate energy costs of various exercises and sports is in Appendix 3.

SECTION B

Food

13

Understanding Food

For a long time in our society the subject of nutrition has been equated with simplistic grade school pictures of the four food groups. We told kids to eat right, but then provided them hot dogs and french fries in the school lunch line. The successful American family has been the one that was so busy that the hamburger stand became the substitute for the dining room.

The only counter to our unhealthy nutrition has been in the area of dieting for weight control. Magazines and tabloids have been built on America's obsession with finding a dietary solution to the fat problem.

Today the whole scene is changing. There is a new interest in nutrition. Junior high and high schools are teaching boys and girls the basics about buying and preparing healthy food. Some of the most popular diet books are really anti-diet books. They advocate careful food planning, the hard work of changing habits, and a much more comprehensive understanding of how, why, and what we eat.

The YMCA has pioneered a sound weight-control program called Slim Living for the past ten years. It is a class that teaches an understanding of the relationship between eating and exercise, a knowledge of basic food values, and a wealth of tips for persons who want to make changes in the way they eat.

YMCA Camp Frost Valley in New Jersey focused the attention of resident camp directors on nutrition and health education in the mid-seventies. Since then YMCA camps across the country have revamped their own kitchens and programs both to teach and to practice good nutrition.

But the real interest in nutrition in America is just beginning to take shape. YMCAs are experiencing tremendous interest in experimental classes on a variety of aspects of healthy eating. The challenge is to help people sort through the flow of new information and apply it to their own lives. The material that follows in this section will become an important text for YMCA classes of the next ten years.

It stands to reason that doctors have always been concerned with what their patients eat and have understood that proper food is vital to good health. Yet not until very recently has there been a significant movement toward making nutrition an area of formal study in medical schools. This was indicated by a 1983 *New York Times* article noting that an increasing number of medical schools were *beginning* to offer instruction in many if not all phases of nutrition. As Dr. August Swanson, director of the Association of Medical Colleges, pointed out: "About 100 of the 143 medical schools in the United States and Canada now offer some sort of courses [in nutrition]."

Even so, most of the courses are electives. According to the *Times* report, only about 15 medical schools had required courses in nutrition.

There is yet another sector of society that one would expect has always been thoroughly immersed in the knowledge of food and how the body uses it: professional sportspeople. Only in the past year or so, however, has nutrition been "discovered" by those whose very business is so intimately allied to good health and physical fitness. In 1983 a major league baseball club and a National Football League team—the Chicago White Sox and the New York Giants—began to use registered nutritionists to advise their players on what and how to eat. In view of the fact that in 1983 the nutrition-conscious White Sox won their division title and for the first time since 1959 had a team in the postseason championship series, one can expect other sports organizations to follow their lead.

A number of pro tennis players, most notably Martina Navratilova, have begun to hire personal nutritionists. After failing to win the 1982 U.S. Open Women's Tennis Singles championship, Navratilova enlisted the aid of Robert Haas, a well-known sports nutritionist. He devised and helped her implement a diet high in carbohydrates and low in fat and protein. The idea was to bring up Martina's energy level. She reduced the fat content of her body to 10 percent, which she felt certain gave her increased stamina, strength, and alertness on the court. Dramatic evidence of this was her victory in the 1983 U.S. Open Women's Tennis Singles and the Virginia Slims Tournament in 1984. Dr. Haas's regimen is outlined in detail in his book *Eat to Win: The Sports Nutrition Bible* (Rawson Associates, 1983).

Furthermore, Miss Navratilova seemed to have lost very little weight and remained the solidly built athlete she had always been. This suggests that good nutrition is not designed solely to trim one's figure, but can simply produce a more efficient, effective physiological system—at least for particular activities.

Developments in the YMCA, in medical groups, and in professional sports all point to the new emphasis on nutrition in our society.

In this section we have sought to bring together the salient information that has been gathered about the chemistry of food. The use of the term "chemistry" is twofold. One facet involves the natural interaction of foods with each other and with our physiologic system; the other is the use of various synthetic chemicals as additives in the manufacture of so many of our foods.

We also want to offer some insights or speculation of a less "scientific" nature that may throw some light on why we eat as we do.

We Are What Our Family Is—and Eats

We have already remarked on the influence of heredity on our essential physical nature. We are tall or short, thickset or slim in good part because of the genes we have inherited from our forebears. The same factor plays a specifically nutritional role. All humans do not have the same number of fat cells; we have more, or less, based on the constitution of our parents, grandparents, and so on. There is no scientific way to count human fat cells, but a look at your relatives is a fairly reliable indicator. If your mother, father, uncles, aunts tend to be heavy with fat, and they do not exercise or eat in ways that promote a leaner body, then you most likely have the same physiological makeup and *the potential* to be fat. You can't reduce the number of fat cells inherent in your body, but if you do not want to accept the genetic fate that has befallen you, you can keep them smaller by controlling how much and what you eat.

To change eating habits, though, is not all that simple. It can entail an emotionally difficult break with your sociocultural "inheritance." We form our eating habits very early in life, at the family table, and well after we leave home we often continue to eat certain foods in certain quantities prepared in certain ways and even at certain speeds because we developed those habits in our most formative years. What's more, to do so reflects or recalls family and/or ethnic traditions by which we gain a sense of emotional stability or solace. There is nothing at all wrong with this except that the food involved (and the amount of it, its style of preparation, and the pace at which it is taken) may not be especially good for us. Or it may have an effect contrary to a new or different attitude about our health and physical condition.

Comedian Buddy Hackett has a story in his repertoire that highlights the point, albeit with some show-business license to exaggerate a bit. He recalls that for the first twenty years of his life he always had a "fire" in his stomach, a burning sensation he assumed was as intrinsic to his existence as the blood running in his veins. Then he went into the army, and after a week of basic training the "fire" went out. At first he was frightened, until he realized it was because he was no longer eating the doughy breads and starchy foods that were the regular fare in his Jewish home in Brooklyn.

Hackett had a revelation. He liked not having a "fire" in the pit of his stomach. He did not entirely give up favorite foods that were part of his family/ethnic tradition, but he did modify his intake of them. Surely, people of all descents can relate to Hackett's tale and tell their own.

A family's economic background is another factor that influences eating habits. Perhaps your parents knew the hard times of the Great Depression of the 1930s, for example, when many people had to eat food that was inexpensive and filling, food that produces longer-lasting energy economically because it takes longer to digest and therefore staves off the feeling of hunger for an extra hour or so. A steady diet of such food, which is high in carbohydrates and fats—whole milk, eggs, cheese, white bread, potatoes, macaroni, cereals, the cheaper cuts of meat—causes overweight, especially when there is not enough offsetting exercise. The point here is, you presently may be eating more fattening food than you need only out of habit developed from a requirement that no longer exists in your current economic circumstances. You may be an unwitting victim of the Depression-Days Eating Syndrome.

Then, too, your choice of foods may be the result of quirks in your family's cookery. Perhaps your mother (or father) did not trust to the cleanliness of food bought at the market and felt it had to be boiled long and hard to be rid of contaminants. There have been more than a few anecdotes told of broccoli and cauliflower and spinach brought to table after a half hour in a pot of water at high bubble that was soggy, lifeless, totally unappetizing.

Little wonder so many children would not "eat their greens," and as adults may still not. On the other hand, many of us have discovered that such vegetables as broccoli, cauliflower, and spinach, when eaten raw or after brief cooking in the stir-fry style of Chinese cuisine, are a pleasure to eat. Needless to say, when eaten this way they also provide a full measure of excellent nutrition that is not poured down the kitchen sink drain.

Food as a Band-Aid

Many professionals in the mental health field assert that people often eat—overeat, actually—to compensate for emotional insecurity, frustration, anxiety, boredom. These conclusions are generally accepted as being on the mark; indeed, few of us probably need a trained psychologist or psychiatrist to tell us what we have observed ourselves. Symbolically, eating gives a feeling of security.

But eating also has a real physiological effect. The very act of eating uses energy, so the more we eat, the more tired (or relaxed) we become. Our arousal level is brought down; we become quiet, less tense. The fundamental problem with gorging oneself with food to allay emotional pain, though, is that a pound of nutritious green beans does not get the job done. A pint of ice cream does, because it tastes better. The personal problem may go away, but only for a while, and what remains is a fat body. The only way to avoid this is to exercise regularly. If this is not done, there comes a time when one cannot work off obesity, not because of laziness, which is a mental attitude, but because the body is unable to do sustained work. It is a downward spiral that can lead to organic illness. Using food to alleviate problems in a career, marriage, whatever, is but a "Band-Aid" that covers the wound but does not eliminate it and can eventually make everything worse.

14

The "Stuff" of Food: Calories, Protein, Carbohydrates, Fats

Becoming aware of social and cultural influences on eating habits is not merely a nostalgia trip. It can point us in a new direction. And to understand that overeating is not always a response to the real needs of the body is to take a step toward finding a true solution to the difficulty. But all of this is of little consequence in helping us take effective action if we do not fully comprehend the essential components of food and how they work. In this respect, of course, there is substantial verifiable evidence, for science has served us exceptionally well through research.

Calories

"Calorie" is perhaps the most commonly referred to term in the average person's nutrition vocabulary. It may also be the most misinterpreted. Contrary to what you may have thought (and what it seems to be when spoken of), *a calorie is not something you eat* as such. Calorie is a term for a measure of heat, which translates into energy. There is a *small calorie,* which is used in physics and chemistry, and the *large calorie* in nutrition, which is noted as a "kcal" because it is equivalent to 1,000 of the small calories. We will use the nutritional "calorie."

A calorie represents an amount of food that produces enough heat/ energy to raise the temperature of 1 kilogram of water 1 degree centigrade (or 4 pounds of water 1 degree Fahrenheit). Our bodies "burn" food calories to energize all our physical actions—from splitting a log for the fireplace to blinking an eye. Our "engines" run on calories oxidized from food, but the "miles-per-gallon" rating is not uniform. It depends on what model of "car" you are—that is, your size, age, sex—and the nature of the activity.

For everyone, the more vigorous the activity, the more calories that are burned. However, men burn more calories than women because they are, on average, heavier and have a greater muscle mass to move. Older people—men *and* women—require fewer calories than younger people because they are generally less active, and their basal metabolism is slower.

A simplified daily calorie requirement for normally active people is as follows:

Age	Men (154 lbs.)	Women (128 lbs.)	Boys (134 lbs.)	Girls (117 lbs.)
25	2,900 calories	2,100 calories		
45	2,600 calories	1,900 calories		
65	2,200 calories	1,600 calories		
15–18			3,400 calories	2,300 calories

If you burn as many calories as you take in, you will not gain or lose weight. If you take in more than you use, you gain weight (and vice versa), which of course is the central problem in most modern-day urban/suburban and even some agricultural environments; we make more deposits in our calorie bank than withdrawals.

Elsewhere on these pages we present a comprehensive chart listing the number of calories present in normal portions of the most commonly used foods—and some uncommonly used ones, too—plus how much one should perform of various exercises to burn them off.

Just about everything we consume during the normal course of our lives—except water and black coffee—contains calories. One food will have more calories than another based on which of the three great classes of nutrients is most prominent in it. The three great classes of nutrients are proteins, carbohydrates, and fats. They are far and away the most abundant nutrients in foods and are so important that even a minimal understanding of nutrition is impossible without a basic knowledge of them.

Protein

Protein is made up of carbon, hydrogen, and oxygen, as are the other two primary nutrients. But protein is the only one containing nitrogen, which is one reason why it is perhaps the most indispensable. Indeed, the word "protein" comes from the Greek for "primary, holding first place." Nitrogen is what makes proteins, which are the "building blocks" of your body.

While protein is present in all living matter, including nonfoods, the human body does not store this nutrient as it does carbohydrates and fats. Nor does the body manufacture much of its own protein. Therefore, the minimum amount of protein required to maintain health is relatively high, it must be steady, and it must be derived from the foods we eat.

Proteins are a source of energy, and they contribute certain valuable minerals and vitamins, but their most important function in nutrition is to build new body tissue and maintain or repair old body tissue. If they have a protein-poor diet, children will not grow fully or properly, and adults will suffer physical deterioration. It is for this reason that any weight-loss diet that substantially eliminates protein-rich food is very ill advised: a protein-poor diet can be extremely dangerous. For instance, there is a disease called kwashiorkor that takes the lives of young children in Asia, Africa, and other parts of the world where the diet is almost exclusively made up of starch foods, such as cassava, corn, and rice, and very little protein.

You can get sufficient protein every day if you eat one average serving of meat, fish, or poultry, a pint of milk, and one to two servings of other protein-rich food. Typical foods that are a good source of protein are lean meat, poultry, fish, dairy products, nuts, peas, beans, whole grains.

The best quality protein, though, is derived from animal foods. Most of the proteins derived from vegetables are not as efficient in sustaining body tissue and have to be consumed in certain combinations to provide optional protein intake. Be sure you know what and how to eat in this way if you are contemplating going on a vegetarian regimen. Of course, protein from animal sources is more expensive, but mixing a small portion of protein-rich animal food with vegetables produces quite ample nutrition. Good examples of this are spaghetti with meat or clam sauce, chili con carne, and most "classic" American sandwiches.

Carbohydrates

The carbohydrate gets its name from its elements—carbon, hydrogen, and oxygen—the suffix *hydrates* deriving from the fact that the hydrogen and oxygen are present in the same two-to-one proportion as in water.

All food carbohydrates are either sugars (*simple* sugars inherent to the foodstuffs) or more complex compounds such as starch and cellulose. Except for lactose (milk sugar), carbohydrates come from fruits and vegetables and from grains, which are particularly desirable.

Carbohydrate-rich foods serve three main purposes in the diet: (1) economical energy, because the foods are relatively the least expensive to produce; (2) some protein, along with vitamins and minerals, although if you want to eat very little or no meat and still fulfill your daily requirement of complete protein, you must eat considerably more grain products and in combinations such as beans and rice and milk and cereal, or eat soybean products such as bean curd; (3) flavor, which comes from the sugars, both simple and refined, that is added in the manufacture of many foods or sprinkled over breakfast cereal, for example. In general, carbohydrates (and fats) are primary fuel nutrients, while protein is the "building block."

There are no definite dietary requirements for carbohydrates, nor any particular level of intake that assures good health. Some peoples around the world eat more carbohydrate-rich food than do others because they may be more readily available and/or are less costly than protein- and fat-rich foods such as meat. However, there is no health hazard in subsisting chiefly on carbohydrate-rich food, *so long as the diet is not completely lacking in protein, fats, minerals, and vitamins.*

In Japan about 80 percent of the population's entire energy intake is made up of carbohydrate (in the form of rice). By contrast, in the United States, with a much greater landmass that allows the raising of great quantities of beef, Americans use more protein- and fat-rich foods; only about half, maybe even less, of their energy derives from carbohydrates. Then again, low-income groups in North America and Europe generally eat a lot of potatoes and bread, as these carbohydrate-rich foods are relatively inexpensive. Thus it is vital that the bread be made from whole grains; or that the popular white bread be enriched during the manufacture with minerals and vitamins that are removed from the highly milled flour used (most white breads are indeed so fortified or "enriched").

Typical carbohydrate-rich foods are corn, peas, rice, carrots, onions, grain cereals, macaroni, bread, and potatoes. Cookies, cakes, jams, and jellies are high in carbohydrates, due to the refined sugar that is so much part of them. Refined sugar, which is pure carbohydrate, provides only caloric energy and has no other nutritional value because any protein, fat, minerals, or vitamins that were in the source of the sugar—cane and beets—are removed in the manufacturing process and not put back.

Fats

Fat is distinguished from carbohydrates and protein by consisting of large amounts of carbon and hydrogen, but a relatively small amount of oxygen. Because of the low oxygen content, the compound oxidizes more quickly and therefore more energy is released. Fat takes the form of a fatty acid, or glycerin, and has a very high fuel value for humans.

Because fat is such a concentrated source of energy, not much of it is necessary in any one meal to prepare you for the day's activity. This is one reason why bacon, in particular the fattier variety that comes from porkbelly and is the most commonly used (Canadian back-bacon is much less fatty and more expensive), has become a standard breakfast food, especially in summer, when we like to eat lighter meals. Bacon gives a lot of energy in a small package. Furthermore, because fat has a high satiety value and does not break down quickly during the digestive process, you can go without eating again for a longer time. However, we often eat more strips of bacon or other fatty food than we need because fat also gives food a flavor we like. This is why eggs fried in butter, for instance, are preferred to those cooked in a specially coated nonstick pan.

Bacon and fried eggs are but a couple of examples expressing the particularly American penchant for fatty foods, a penchant that may stem at least in part from the fact that the cost of such foods in the United States is quite reasonable compared to their cost in many other parts of the world. To be able to eat it in quantity, then, is a reflection of the American Dream of plenty come true, and seems to symbolize the success of our economic system. In this sense, eating a big steak becomes a form of self-congratulation. Then again, in the Middle Ages it was felt that meat made one stupid and melancholy. In *Twelfth Night* Shakespeare wrote, "I am a greater eater of beef, and I believe that does harm to my wit."

In any event, nutritionists feel that a diet for the average person living in a temperate climate should include about 25 percent fat. Surveys indicate the average American has 40 percent fat in his diet.

Fat deposits in the body can be advantageous *if they are moderate.* Fat just under the skin and around the abdominal area constitutes a reserve store of energy that can be called on when needed. These fat deposits also support organs, protecting them from injury, and prevent an undue loss of body heat because fat is a poor conductor of heat. It is because of this that Eskimos are able to live where they do, and it is the only reason their diet, or that of anyone else living in the Arctic, is about 75 percent fat.

What's more, because of its acid nature, fat is necessary to break down foods so their nutrients can be released into the blood system. Indeed, a totally fat-free diet will cause poor growth or physical degeneration, just as a lack of protein will, plus skin problems such as eczema, and other illnesses. It is especially important that infants have a generous supply of fat delivered through their food; milk is the usual way.

As for adults, there is some fat in just about everything eaten, so overeating in general—eating more than activity uses—means storing an excess. The added weight puts a strain on the heart and other vital organs. Insurance company figures indicate that overweight persons have a much lower life-expectancy rate than those who maintain normal weight for their height and age.

SATURATED FAT/UNSATURATED FAT AND CHOLESTEROL

Basically, there are two kinds of fat, saturated and unsaturated. A saturated fat is so called because all the hydrogen bonds in its molecular structure are filled. As its name implies, saturated fat is somewhat thicker than its opposite number. This is born out by the fact that it is solid at room temperature. Butter is the most notable example of a saturated fat. Otherwise, it is generally a part of the foodstuff that contains it. It is more or less hidden from view, or at least is not obvious (except in steak marbled with fat), which can make it difficult to detect and avoid if you're cutting down intake.

Saturated fat comes primarily from animal food and food products. Some plant foods contain saturated fat, coconut in particular, but generally not enough to be important. The most common "carriers" of saturated fat are beef, mutton, pork, veal, poultry, bacon, eggs, cheeses, whole milk, herring, and salmon. Beef has the highest proportion.

Unsaturated fat has some unfilled hydrogen bonds; the polyunsaturates have a couple more unfilled. These derive from the vegetable kingdom and tend to be in liquid form at room temperature. They are generally the oils used in cooking. Peanut and olive oil are unsaturated; corn, soybean, cottonseed, and safflower oil are polyunsaturated.

An increasing number of nutritionists are recommending a reduced intake of saturated fat because it contains a fattylike substance called cholesterol, which appears only in animals. There has been considerable controversy surrounding cholesterol and the potentially serious effects of having too much of it in the system. The research is far from complete, but there has been enough to warrant a warning about it.

Cholesterol, from the Greek *chole* for "bile" and *sterol* for "solid," is necessary in the body. It aids the digestive process, is used in making sex hormones, and has a number of other important functions. The body makes its own cholesterol, and usually enough for its purposes. The problem arises when we eat foods that contain cholesterol. The combination of endogenous and exogenous cholesterol raises the total level, or count, in the system. An excess of cholesterol in the bloodstream combines with other substances to form scaly deposits known as plaques that stick to and build up on the walls of the arteries. The arteries eventually narrow, so the flow of blood through them becomes restricted. This "plugging" of the arteries, in medical terminology called *atherosclerosis,* can in time lead to a reduced blood flow to the heart and by a different mechanism damage some portion of the heart muscle. The result is a heart attack.

Some definitive research pointing to this conclusion includes the use of laboratory rabbits. The rabbits were fed large amounts of cholesterol, which is foreign to these vegetarians, and atherosclerosis was induced. There have also been surveys indicating that levels of cholesterol in the system tend to be higher, and heart disease more common, in more prosperous nations where animal fats are eaten in quantity.

As noted, none of the negative theories about cholesterol has been proven beyond the shadow of a doubt. Other studies of the substance have found that there is considerable variation in the cholesterol count of normal individuals, no matter what their diet is. Some people have a very high *natural* (endogenous) cholesterol level—they make more than do others—and don't seem to suffer the supposed effects, even though they also take in more through food. Some have much less cholesterol, and it is conceivable that such individuals could, and perhaps should, eat as many eggs as they like.

It has also been found that pectin seems to lower the cholesterol level in the body. Pectin is a water-soluble carbohydrate derivative found in many fruits; it is the basis of most jellies. One study showed that 15 grams of pectin a day over a three-week period reduced the serum cholesterol level in nine of fifteen subjects by 15 percent. This suggests that eating an apple a day may indeed keep the doctor away.

Your cholesterol level can be definitively measured. According to the American Heart Association, a person with 250 milligrams or more of cholesterol per 100 milliliters of blood runs about three times the risk of heart attack than a person with a cholesterol count below 200 milligrams.

When food manufacturers advertise polyunsaturated products, they often imply that their use reduces, if not eliminates, the risk of heart attack (or stroke). They may be wrong, they may be right, they may be somewhere in between. We cannot say one way or another, but based on what has been learned to date about cholesterol, the YMCA thinks it prudent to eat less saturated fat. If nothing else, you will help yourself avoid obesity.

15

Vitamins

During the great voyages of discovery in the fifteenth century many sailors suffered from scurvy, the symptoms of which include bleeding of the gums, loosening of the teeth, anemia, and general debility. More than half of Vasco da Gama's crew died from scurvy on his first trip around the Cape of Good Hope. In 1747 a Scots naval surgeon named James Lind treated scurvy-ridden sailors with lemons and oranges and got curative results immediately. Two years later the British navy made lime juice part of regular rations during long voyages, and scurvy was largely eliminated. It was for this reason that British sailors came to be called *limeys*. Of course, the citrus that Lind fed the sailors contained vitamin C, which had been lacking in their diet and probably was not taken aboard because in its natural state the fruit did not keep very long. Modern transportation and food preserving methods have made scurvy practically nonexistent at sea and rare on land.

Dr. Lind was apparently working on a hunch in treating scurvy, because the scientific discovery of vitamins did not occur until the early 1900s, when an English biochemist named Frederick Gowland Hopkins (later, *Sir* Frederick) fed laboratory rats a diet of pure protein, fat, and carbohydrates and saw them sicken and die. By adding less than one third of a teaspoonful of milk per day to the same highly purified diet, Hopkins' next group of rats lived on in good health. His conclusion was that an essential organic substance, previously unknown, existed in foods in their natural state and were absolutely essential to life (in the case of his laboratory rats it was vitamins A and C). In other words, humans had been eating—or not eating—vitamins long before they realized it. Hopkins received a share of the 1929 Nobel Prize for

Physiology and Medicine for his work, which was the discovery of what he initially called "accessory food factors" and later the vitamin.

Since then, thirteen vitamins have been isolated. There may be more discovered at any time. (However, all vitamins can be manufactured synthetically, and they are as good as the real thing.)

Vitamins do not in themselves supply energy or build and maintain body tissue. What they do is stimulate, or catalyze, the chemical reactions that get the nutrients to do their job. You might say vitamins are the spark that ignites the fuel that runs our "engine" and keeps the engine running smoothly. The human body does not make its own vitamins, as it does cholesterol, say, but very little of any vitamin is required daily—in many cases only a trace amount—and even in the simplest of *balanced* diets you will acquire what is needed.

For all that, many people, usually as they get older, feel they must supplement their vitamin intake. It is relatively inexpensive to buy bottles of vitamin tablets, and it seems harmless enough. However, while in some instances extra vitamins can be useful, such as during the last half of pregnancy and in the lactation period (when women might take vitamin B_2, riboflavin), there has been dramatic evidence that an excess of vitamins can have bad effects. For example, a food faddist in England drank a gallon of vitamin A-rich carrot juice every day over a period of time, turned a bright orange yellow, and died of cirrhosis of the liver. And a recent report in *The New England Journal of Medicine* found that too much vitamin B_6 (commonly sold in health-food stores, used by body builders, and prescribed by some gynecologists for menstrual swelling) can cause peripheral nerve damage. It was found that patients suffering numbness or a loss of sensation improved "gratifyingly" after they stopped taking vitamin B_6, although there was some residual damage.

The YMCA has taken a strong stand against the fad of excessive vitamin supplements. The medical opinion that guides this position is that supplementary vitamin intake is unnecessary and potentially harmful.

The U.S. Food and Drug Administration has formulated a recommended daily allowance (U.S. RDA) of vitamins, minerals, and protein. Since few consumers are likely to carry the complete listing with them to the market, more and more food packagers are presenting on their labels the percentage of vitamins, minerals, and sometimes protein contained in each serving of the particular food. While this may not be the most precise method, it is the best so far devised to advise the general public on vitamin intake in their regular diet. However, the YMCA wants you to know that the U.S. RDA percentages marked on food packages is pegged to the needs determined for adults in normal good health. They may not be suitable for infants, lactating women, and other special cases. The Y recommends that you seek the advice of your doctor on just how much of each vitamin (and mineral and protein) you should take daily.

A table listing the thirteen vitamins, their primary sources in foods, their main roles, deficiency symptoms, and the risks of overdoses is in Appendix 4.

16

Minerals

There are seven essential minerals and nine trace elements, all of which are vital to the proper functioning of the body. Like vitamins, minerals are not primary energy sources, but regulators and catalysts within the physiological system. For example, iron is a key factor in making the hemoglobin that enables the red corpuscles to carry oxygen to, and carbon dioxide from, the tissues. The life of tissue cells is very dependent on this. Pernicious anemia is one result of iron deficiency.

Calcium and phosphorous combined give strength and substance to bones and teeth and are particularly important for growing children, although somewhat less so for adults. That is why kids are told to drink their milk every day—their future well-being is contingent upon it. However, children do not need the extra fat contained in whole milk, especially those with an overweight problem. They will get all the calcium they need from the low-fat milks (skim, 1%, and 2%).

Minerals are inorganic elements—they derive from nonliving sources—and are generally not retained in the body so must be replenished daily. However, only very small amounts are needed and they are all widely distributed in our foods. A balanced diet in any of the world's cuisines practically assures sufficient mineral requirements. But there are no guarantees. A fairly high percentage of teenagers may be deficient in iron, probably because they do not eat enough leafy green vegetables, a rich source of this mineral. Adult women also tend to be iron-deficient. This is believed to be a natural deficiency peculiar to the sex, perhaps due in some part to blood loss through menstruation. In this case, iron supplements can be taken.

Indeed, all the known mineral nutrients (the list is at the end of this chapter) are available in the marketplace in man-made form. But there may be even more question about the viability of taking supplementary mineral pills than about taking vitamin pills. In *Nutrition and Physical Fitness,* Drs. Bogert, Briggs, and Calloway note that all minerals are toxic when overlarge amounts are taken into the body. For example, "About twice the amount of fluorine which provides protection against dental caries will cause mottling of the teeth."

Warnings on bottles that say to keep iron pills and other minerals out of the reach of children further testify to the toxicity of large doses of minerals.

It comes down to a matter of too much of a good thing and striking a balance. The YMCA concurs with Dr. C. G. King, of the Nutrition Foundation, who stresses showing "how urgent the need is for the public as well as scientists to understand the concept that all nutrients are safe or useful to the body within a limited quantitative range."

The seven essential minerals, or macrominerals, are:

    calcium
    phosphorous
    magnesium
    potassium
    sulfur
    chloride
    sodium

The nine trace minerals are:

    iron
    copper
    zinc
    iodine
    fluorine
    chromium
    selenium
    manganese
    molybdenum

A table of minerals providing the primary sources, main roles, deficiency symptoms, and overdose risks is in Appendix 5.

17

Water

Water is second only to oxygen in importance to the body. You can live for weeks without solid food, but only for a few days without water. About 100 pounds of a 150-pound man's weight is in water, which is pertinent to every physiological/chemical process—from carrying nutrients through the bloodstream to all organs and cells to removing waste products. Another function of water that many overlook is in regulating body temperature, which water equalizes by transporting heat from one part to another during the course of circulation.

We need five to six pints of water a day to replace what we lose through breathing, excretion, and perspiration. Our body creates some of that requirement through digestion and metabolism. We take in about two pints with food (virtually all food contains some water, even the driest of crackers, which are about 5 percent water). The rest of the daily quota should come from drinking five to six glasses of water, although not that much need be taken "straight" if your diet includes soup, milk, tea, coffee, or other beverages. On the other hand, much of this other form of water intake includes calories—often many more than needed for maintaining proper weight. The calories in a glass of soda pop (70 to 100 from the sugar) tend to stick around after the water itself has been expelled. The same goes for a 12-ounce bottle of beer (150 calories), a glass of table wine (80 to 120 calories), a mixed drink (1½ ounces of 86-proof Scotch whiskey with water or soda—130 calories), a cup of coffee with cream and sugar (about 45 calories). Plain water and some carbonated "seltzer" waters contain no calories, carbohydrates, protein, or fat, but *do* contain some minerals and vitamins.

Bottled Water

In the past few years there has been a significant increase in the use of commercially bottled "mineral" water, which is taken from deep-underground springs.

This interest is in close conjunction with the concern of many for their general health and weight and the worries about toxic substances getting into tap water via industrial and nuclear-energy waste. There are also those who feel municipal purification of water is inadequate, and that it contains too much chlorination. No one seriously questions the healthiness of the mineral waters, which are not treated (other than with carbonation in some cases), but are they as nutritious as the bottled-water industry would like us to believe?

The assumption is that "mineral" water is not only different from tap water but better for us. Accordingly, the price is higher. The American Waterworks Association has said that one gallon of ordinary municipal tap water costs, on average, a penny, and that the same quantity of any brand of commercial "mineral" water sells for approximately $3.16. Do we get our money's worth in nutrition?

The State of California decided to define mineral water so as to regulate the labeling of all commercial brands sold in the state. A food technology specialist with the California Department of Health Services, Dr. Jack Sheneman, gave the basic definition as "that which contains more than 500 milligrams per liter of totally dissolved solids. That is, if a liter of water allowed to evaporate leaves 1/50 of an ounce or more of minerals, it is mineral water."

By this criterion some bottled waters had to be relabeled to be sold in California. Dr. Sheneman also remarked that the city of Fresno's tap water "happens to contain 540 mgs of minerals," the same amount as the most popular commercial bottled water on the market.

"All basic water has *some* mineral content," said Dr. Sheneman, "so *all* water can be said to be mineral water."

People on a salt-free diet might want to avoid mineral water (the commercial brands), since most of them contain sodium, although the amount is generally low. On the whole, spring water cannot hurt you, but how much it can actually help you is difficult to say because, as Dr. Sheneman pointed out, "they all have different mineral makeups. It depends on what an individual may need. In any case, most mineral nutrition comes from food, because there is no significant amount [of minerals] in water. In terms of nutritional value you get as many valuable minerals from one glass of milk or a hamburger as from *five gallons* of water of any kind."

Dr. Sheneman allowed that the most positive dietary aspect of bottled water is the absence of sugar or other fattening agents, but, he concluded, "tap water doesn't have any, either."

Whatever your water source, it is almost impossible to drink too much in a day—the body will eventually throw off the excess. But some people don't drink enough water, many on the mistaken notion that this is a way to lose weight. Perhaps they confuse the bloated feeling from drinking too much water with weight gain, but as we have shown, water has nothing in it that "sticks to the bones." In fact, water is retained in the body only as required by the tissues or in direct proportion to the amount of tissue. Thus, fat people retain more water because they are fat. This leads to another conventionally held idea about water that is especially risky: thinking you can lose weight by heavy sweating.

No-Sweat Weight Loss

The usual means for trying to lose weight by sweating are sitting in a steam room, sometimes while wearing a rubber "sweat suit," or exercising in such an outfit on warm, humid days. Such practices may take off a pound or two of total body weight, but only in water—not in fat, the real culprit. At that, the weight loss is only temporary—or should be—because the lost water must be replaced very soon to maintain a stable system and avoid the risk of dehydration.

Sitting in a steam room or exercising in an overwarm environment diminishes the body's ability to dispel heat normally. Evaporation of sweat is the main means of heat dissipation at the surface of the skin. If you wear a rubber suit, the heat and sweat given off between the suit and body are trapped, causing body temperature to rise much higher than normal. This puts a great strain on the heat-regulating mechanisms of the body and leads to a loss of too much body water, a decrease in blood volume, a severe rise in body temperature, and possible circulatory collapse and heat stroke. We strongly recommend that rubber suits not be worn at any time in an exercise or weight-loss program.

Water contains no calories so is not fattening. You lose weight by burning calories, not water. To severely limit your intake of water or cause a significant reduction by excessive, unventilated sweating is to court deep trouble. You may without real danger lose all your reserve of carbohydrates and fat and about half your protein, but a loss of 10 percent of total body water is very serious, and a loss of 20 to 22 percent is fatal.

18

Fiber

Fiber is the more up-to-date, quasi-technical term for what many of our parents called "roughage." Either way, it is foods or food components that do not break down in the digestive tract and, as a residue of bulk in the lower abdomen, fosters the comfortable, regular evacuation of fecal matter. Fiber may not be a true nutrient, but it has an excellent, important regulatory function in the system; it makes the use of commercially prepared laxatives unnecessary.

The insoluble fiber that serves as a laxative is essentially cellulose, hemicellulose, or lignin. It is best acquired as an integral part of food, not as something taken separately or mixed with other foods. Bran has been used extensively this way. But adding this highly concentrated source of fiber, which has a coarse quality, to a diet already rich in naturally fibrous food gives no added benefit, and the intestines can be irritated.

Whole grains are a major source of fiber so long as their outercoats are not discarded, such as during the milling of the flour to make white bread. Whole-grain breads retain their nutrients without the need of enrichment *and* provide fiber. A wide variety of other foodstuffs have also been discovered to be good sources of fiber. They include peas, broccoli, and white, kidney, and pinto beans. Also high in fiber are potatoes, carrots, tomatoes, beets, squash, and apples, all of which provide even more fiber if left unpeeled.

A lot of people have always removed the edible outercoats or skins of certain fibrous foods, perhaps because they come from the soil and are perceived to be dirty, or because they make chewing more difficult. But by simply scrubbing a carrot or potato and eating the whole item the food not only has more fiber but provides more of its true nutrients and very often has a better taste.

Indeed, Dr. Peter Van Soest, professor of animal nutrition at Cornell University and a leading fiber researcher, has found that cooking techniques that tend to enhance the flavor of foods can also increase their fiber content. Stir-frying vegetables in the Chinese style is one example. Dr. Soest also notes that sautéed vegetables have more fiber than boiled vegetables, although sautéing them in butter raises the cholesterol and caloric level of your meal. Steaming food removes less fiber than boiling. Pureeing vegetables reduces their fiber content, and turning fruit into juice leaves almost no fiber at all. And without any more preparation than putting them out in a bowl, strawberries and blackberries are very high in fiber.

The New York Times reported recently of some studies indicating that fiber may be useful in weight reduction. Eating a diet of high-fiber foods appears to be more satisfying than a meal made up of meats, dairy products, and desserts, with their greater amounts of fat and simple carbohydrates. The high-fiber diet contains fewer calories, but takes up more space in the stomach, absorbs water, slows down digestion, and makes one feel satiated longer.

There has also been research leading scientists to believe the so-called soluble fibers—gums, pectins, and mucilages—found in many fruits and vegetables may help to stabilize the level of sugar in the blood and lower the levels of fat and cholesterol. Finally, Dr. James Anderson, chief of endocrinology at the University of Kentucky Medical Center, has been using a diet high in soluble fibers to treat diabetes.

A list of commonly used foods and their fiber content is in Appendix 6.

19

Salt

The time has arrived when people sit down to a meal *without* automatically sprinkling salt in their soup or salad or entrée *before* tasting a morsel. They don't even notice the absence of a salt shaker on the table.

In a word, there has been an increasing awareness that most of us have been using too much salt in our diet, a practice that appears to be modifying. Even food manufacturers, from whom we get so much of our extra salt, have begun producing and advertising "salt-free," "low-salt," "no salt added" tomato sauce, cottage cheese, canned soups and vegetables, and crackers.

Nothing could make doctors happier. The compound sodium chloride (table salt) is a vital constituent of the human body. It is the principal regulator of the balance of water and dissolved substances outside the cells. But an excess of salt can have a deleterious effect. The more salt you take in, the more liquid you must drink to dissolve the sodium. (It is not out of pure generosity that tavernkeepers put out bowls of pretzels, peanuts, and other salty tidbits for their customers.) If over a period of time more sodium is taken in than can be excreted, the retained sodium holds water in the body and blood volume rises. This causes the blood vessels to contract so that more blood has to pass through narrower channels. Blood pressure increases and can eventually lead to hypertension.

Excess sodium also increases the amount of water in and around the body tissues. This results in swelling, or edema. If the swelling occurs around the heart, the result can be congestive heart failure.

Research has clearly established the link between excessive consumption of sodium and high blood pressure (hypertension), as well as its link with heart ailments, kidney disease, and stroke. The typical American diet is rich in sodium, and an estimated 34 million Americans suffer from hypertension, making it one of the nation's most widespread health problems. Hypertension is a leading cause of death and disability in Japan, another heavy user of salt. (The rate is even higher in northern Japan, where the most salt is consumed in that country.)

Some people hold the view that hypertension is largely a psychological problem endemic to fast-paced modern urban cultures. However, *New York Times* nutrition writer Jane Brody has pointed out that high blood pressure is common among the Gashgai nomads of southern Iran, where such pressures do not exist but *where a lot of salt is consumed.* Finally, a Mayo Clinic study has shown that sodium restriction alone can lower blood pressure to normal in persons with mild hypertension.

Salt has been prized by man for many hundreds of years. An esteemed person is the "salt of the earth." The word "salary" stems from the custom in ancient Rome of paying soldiers in rations of salt (*sal*). But it appears the *craving* for salt is not based on real need. Enough sodium is naturally present in enough foods and water to meet normal requirements. Dr. Lot Page, a specialist in hypertension, has concluded after an extensive study of salt in the diet of pre-Industrial Age peoples that "salt appetite is determined by early dietary habits."

The salt habit may well have begun in earnest in the days before refrigeration, when salt was used extensively to preserve foods. For that matter, salt, usually in combination with other chemicals, is still used as a food preservative. Of course, salt also increases or develops the flavor in foods. But it appears that the taste is an acquired one. Dr. Marilyn Fregley, a behavioral scientist at the University of Florida, has noted that when a Bolivian hunting tribe was first introduced to salt by an American, they did not like the taste, and only after more use was a craving for it developed. Jane Brody has cited evidence that newborn babies "grimace when given something salty to taste" and that an infant does not eat less of low- or no-salt strained foods. But because so much salt is added to baby food, the taste becomes fixed, which is reflected by a study showing that preschool children preferred a salted beef stew over an unsalted one. And of course, children are very fond of salty snacks. (It should be noted that the suggested RDA for children is much lower than for adults, and that baby-food makers have begun to eliminate or at least reduce the amount of salt in their products.)

The physiological requirement for sodium has been put at 220 milligrams a day—$1/10$ of a teaspoon of salt. The RDA is much higher, 1,100 to 3,300 mgs per day, for adults—3 to 8 grams, or about 1 teaspoonful. But Americans average around $3\frac{1}{2}$ teaspoons of salt daily.

Dr. Mark Hegsted, of the Human Nutrition Center of the U.S.

Department of Agriculture, has said that the current level of salt intake by Americans is halfway to the toxic level, and he has suggested that "if salt were a new food additive, it is doubtful that it would be classified as safe and certainly not [safe] at the level most of us consume [it]."

It is not so much that we are too liberal with the salt shaker at the table; we simply compound the problem in this way. About two thirds of our salt intake is from processed foods, which accounts for 55 percent of what Americans eat. A startling example is the fact that 3½ ounces of fresh garden peas contain only 2 mgs of sodium, whereas the same serving of canned peas has 236 mgs. And there are 4 mgs of sodium in six spears of fresh asparagus, but 410 mgs in six canned spears. When preparing canned vegetables, strain off the canning juice and rinse the vegetables in water to eliminate as much salted fluid as you can.

You can expect such fermented foods as bottled pickles and sauerkraut to be laden with sodium, which is used as a preservative. One analysis has shown that one large kosher dill pickle from a bottle contains 1,137 mgs of sodium—that is a third of the maximum RDA. The sodium content of some processed foods is surprising in another way. Who would imagine that an ounce of cornflakes would have twice the amount of sodium as an ounce of cocktail peanuts? But this is so—260 mgs to 132 mgs. Or that two slices of white bread would have more sodium than an ounce of potato chips? Analysis has shown this, too—234 mgs to 191 mgs.

Why do food processors put so much sodium in their products? Because it's the least expensive way to increase the flavor of food and to obtain longer shelf life. Perhaps with enough consumer resistance clearly attributable to excessive salt content, food processors will be forced to find new and better ways to prepare their products for the market.

There has been some use of potassium chloride as a substitute for people on a salt-free diet. But Dr. Jean Mayer warns that some people cannot tolerate increased amounts of potassium, and for this reason he recommends the use of any potassium salt only with a doctor's consent. In any case, as Dr. Mayer notes, salt substitutes do not taste like real salt. One must acquire a taste for them, and then they may be as overwhelming as excessive sodium chloride often is, burying the natural flavor of the foods in which they are used.

The best substitute for table salt is the creative use of herbs and spices as food flavorings. In this respect, the American Heart Association has issued a list suggesting ways for you to season different foods without the use of salt. That list is in Appendix 7.

20

Sugar

Refined sugar is easily the most used food *additive* we eat. The latest statistics show that the average American eats around 128 pounds of sugar a year. To put that figure in closer perspective, it amounts to about a third of a pound of sugar a day. Again, as with salt, the greatest portion of our sugar intake comes to us through processed foods. Within that category, the two with the most are sweetened soft drinks and candy bars. A 12-ounce bottle of soda pop contains anywhere from 6 to 9 teaspoons of sugar. A 1-ounce chocolate bar contains 6 teaspoons.

Refined sugar by itself has no nutritional value whatsoever. It provides only calories, or energy. A soft drink—sugar mixed with water, basically—is simply a bottle of "empty calories." A candy bar will have some nutrients (in the chocolate, nuts, etc.), but hardly enough to sustain anyone for very long.

But many of our basic, nutritional foods that contain natural sugar also have refined sugar added in their processing. For instance, in every tablespoon of catsup there is a teaspoon of sugar. Sugar is also processed into crackers, breads, soups, bouillon cubes, cured meats, salad dressings, spaghetti sauces, and, of course, just about every dessert or between-meals snack we eat. The labels on these foods may not say they contain sugar, specifically, because it comes in different forms. For the most part the ingredient has an *-ose* suffix, as in fructose (fruit sugar), lactose (milk sugar), and maltose (malt sugar), but it might also be "hidden" under the designation of corn syrup, maple syrup, honey, or molasses. Look for these on labels.

Food processors use sugar to help food retain moisture, to prevent spoilage, and to improve texture and appearance. But its overriding aim is to flavor the food. There is nothing new in this. Stone Age man had a sweet tooth, which was satisfied with honey. Sugarcane was an important product in India around 5000 B.C. A number of great fortunes were made by satisfying man's love of sweets, especially when modern methods of refining the confection were developed and sugar was made available at a reasonable cost to the average consumer. It would seem this was when sugar became a "problem" food. We don't know whether enough sugar was eaten in early times to cause the illnesses now associated with it, but by the end of the nineteenth century in the United States sugar was "on its way."

All the facts are not yet in regarding the various illnesses claimed to be caused by an excess of sugar in the diet, but no one questions that tooth decay is one of them. Bacteria in the mouth combine with sugar to form an acid that slowly but inexorably wears away tooth enamel. However, there is evidence that if sugar is eaten with meals, and especially if teeth are brushed or the mouth is rinsed out with water within fifteen minutes after the meal, the incidence of tooth decay is reduced. It is sugary snacks, especially the gooey ones, between meals that bring dental bills.

No one can say with certainty what causes diabetes—the "sugar disease"—but obesity seems to be one, and people who eat too much sugar and not enough nutritious food and/or do not exercise enough, get fat. Some doctors think heart disease can result from a steady overdose of sugar, but there has not yet been enough research done on this. What is more, it cannot be said that sugar itself makes people fatter than do other carbohydrates or fats. But because sugar is such a highly concentrated form of energy and is so easily combined with other foods, it is easy to eat it in quantity, especially since it tastes so good. Furthermore, sugar does not fill people up as "real" food does. Therefore, people who eat too much of it and add huge amounts of calories to their diet get no *sense* that they must exercise to work them off, and obesity more or less sneaks up on them.

The idea that eating a lot of sugar does *not* stimulate the desire to exercise seems contrary to a long-held notion that sugar is a source of "quick energy" to spark activity. A "shot" of sugar will indeed set you going, but the spurt lasts a very short time—a matter of minutes—and can be followed by a greater letdown. That's because as soon as the blood sugar rises from the sugar intake, your pancreas begins to bring it back down with secretions of insulin. You would need an enormous quantity of sugar to stay on an energy "high" for any length of time. In either case, the sugar-induced "pick-me-up" that is quickly put down—

what Dr. Kenneth Cooper calls the Yo-Yo Effect—can cause dizziness, light-headedness, and possibly even fainting.

The Yo-Yo Effect also quashes another old notion about sugar: that it reduces appetite. The quick rise and fall in blood sugar actually can leave you hungrier.

It seems clear that the negative effects—real or potential—of sugar so outweigh the positive that we should all put a permanent seal on our private sugar bowl and buy fewer processed foods containing a high—or any—level of sugar. That is not likely to happen, but surely there can be a substantial reduction in sugar intake by, let's say, eating more fresh fruit for desserts and snacks, instead of ice cream and cake. Then the occasional sugar spree of a banana split or chocolate éclair becomes an *occasion,* a bit of fun.

21

The "Other" Chemicals in Food

Probably the biggest controversy revolving around nutrition and the food industry in recent times is the use of chemicals in processed foodstuffs. The subject has generated much scientific research, extensive coverage through magazine and newspaper articles, books, and television, and it has stirred considerable debate and official hearings within the government leading to legislative action. At least one commercial by-product of all this has been the impressive growth of the "health food" business, which we will discuss. But most important, the average person has become far more conscious than ever before of what is in the food he/she eats every day.

From the overall tone of the argument it would seem you must be on either one side of the issue or the other—for or against chemicals in our food. Of course, it is not that simple. Strictly speaking, since our basic foods originate in the earth, they *are* chemicals. But that is to beg the question. The debate swirls around the chemicals that are *added* to food—the "other" chemicals.

In many cases, these are natural products of the earth. Indeed, the two chemical additives that constitute by far the highest percentage of use are "naturals"—sugar and salt. Figures indicate that of the 1,500 pounds of food the average American eats per year, 152 pounds of it is chemical additives. And of that, 128 pounds of sugar; 15 pounds is salt. The remaining 9 pounds include synthetic reproductions of nature's work, and some wholly man-made, artificial substances that are not found in nature.

The essential question is, are these chemicals safe to eat? But the most urgent question within that question is, do they cause cancer? This applies primarily to synthetic and artificial substances. We cannot make a definitive judgment, any more than the experts can who devote themselves exclusively to the matter of chemical safety. It can be noted, though, that while the first Food and Drugs Act prohibiting the adulteration of processed foods with toxic ingredients was passed in 1906, it wasn't until 1958 that the law required that new food chemicals be shown to be safe *before* they could be added to foods. Since that time certain additives have been banned as unsafe. They include two artificial sweeteners (dulcin and cyclamate), a beer foam stabilizer (cobalt sulfate), and three coloring agents.

Our intention here is to present an overview of the additive issue. We will present, too, a list of the chemicals most often used, their description and purpose, and brief comments and suggestions on their use.

No chemical can be said to be absolutely safe to consume, and certainly not if taken in sizable amounts. This, by the way, brings up one of the central arguments of food industry spokespeople regarding the testing of additives. These tests are necessarily done on laboratory animals. In order to have a correlation to humans, the amount of an additive given the animals is generally very large. The food industry feels this is not a fair way to indicate how the additive will actually affect humans, who will receive far, far smaller doses. There are other uncertain aspects about testing procedures, but they go beyond the scope of this book. For our purposes, the remarks made here are on the assumption that the chemical additives in our food are within acceptable limits.

Over four hundred additives have been considered safe to consume and given the designation GRAS—Generally Recognized as Safe—by the Food and Drug Administration. However, the designation is not carved in stone. An artificial coloring used in hot dogs, Orange B, was approved by the FDA in 1966, but in 1978 the manufacturer of the additive stopped making it after finding it contained a cancer-causing impurity. More recently, the sweetener saccharin was removed from the GRAS list.

Most GRAS substances serve a worthy purpose. Some make food more nutritious. Sulfites increase the stability of vitamin C; sulfur dioxide preserves vitamin C and beta carotene; ascorbic acid prevents iron and copper from damaging vitamins A, E, thiamin, and folic acid. In some instances the additives only restore the nutrients that were lost at an early stage in the processing; we have cited white bread as one such, and another staple "enriched" with vitamins is white rice. Then there is calcium propionate, an additive that keeps bread from getting moldy before two or three days and also provides a valuable nutrient—calcium. Ironically, while calcium propionate has been proven quite safe, some breadmakers have been eliminating it, presumably to attract the "natural food" enthusiast with a "no preservatives added" product.

Additives used as preservatives are a factor in holding down the cost of food. Because there is less fear of spoilage over a significant length of time, such foods can be produced in very large and thereby more economical quantities. There is also another social implication. Foods with preservatives added to them can be stocked up, precluding the need for frequent shopping and, in many cases, for time-consuming food preparation.

A good many additives are used for cosmetic purposes; that is, to give foods a certain texture and/or color believed to be more appealing. The most controversial additives seem to be in this category. It is also the case that many, if not all, foods with artificial colorings have very little nutritional value; they tend to be soda pop, candy, and other "junk foods." With enough information to go by, the decision as to whether these additives are really necessary and their results really desirable should be made by the consumer. With that in mind we offer descriptions of the additives most used in our food in Appendix 8.

22

"Health"/"Organic-Natural" Foods

The concern over chemicals added to food when it is being processed for the market is compounded by the application of chemical fertilizers and pesticides on or around a steer, a stand of wheat, or a carrot, before they are ready for the butcher, the baker, or the canner. The combination has spawned the multibillion-dollar "health" food industry. But despite its reassuring sound, "health" food is also controversial.

What *is* "health" food? Basically, its advocates define it as that which is free of chemical additives and has been grown without the use of synthetic chemical fertilizers and pesticides. Fertilizers used are those that "occur naturally," such as animal manure, worm castings, hay that has been plowed back into the earth. This is also the definition of "organic" food, which is also referred to as "natural" food. All three are pretty much synonymous. Advocates of health food insist that what they eat is healthier.

Skeptics define health food as anything sold in a health food store. But they go much further than a quip in denying the primary health food claims. Noted nutrition educator Dr. Ruth Leverton was speaking for the U.S. Department of Agriculture's Agricultural Research Service when she said: "The type of fertilizer used is not a determining factor in the nutrition of a plant."

In other words, the scientific fact is that carrots will have a lot of vitamin A and all other components and characteristics of the specie because of their genetic structure, which no fertilizer can change. Carrots may be bigger or smaller, and there may be more or less of them in a crop, depending on the quality of the soil in which they are grown, but they will still be carrots.

As the FDA's Dr. Charles C. Edwards has said, "The most sophisticated techniques of chemical analysis have not detected any difference between *organic* and *ordinary* food."

Are health foods safer to eat, then? Dr. Jean Mayer, a highly respected authority on food and nutrition, has said: "Organic foods may escape chemical pollution, but biologically speaking they tend to be the most contaminated of all. Organic fertilizers of animal origin are conspicuously the most likely to contain gastrointestinal parasites. In fact, in many underdeveloped areas widespread infections have been eliminated decisively by switching from age-old (organic) fertilizing methods to chemical fertilizers.

"I am constantly astonished to find that more and more young people believe the only reason for washing fruits and vegetables to be consumed raw is to eliminate pesticides. Apparently they have forgotten that the major danger in eating is still preeminently bacterial or parasitic contamination."

The health food advocates' fear of pesticides is not unwarranted. At the same time, it is estimated that without pesticides crop losses would mean a very substantial rise in the cost of basic foodstuffs. What's more, pesticide control may be even more closely monitored by government agencies than food additives, and some have been banned, DDT being the most notorious one.

Proponents of health food might be on firmer ground if they dropped the insistence on the nutritional superiority of organically grown food and rested their case on diet itself. The fresh, unadulterated peanut butter sold in health food stores (and now in some supermarkets), with the peanuts ground right before your eyes, is indeed excellent. Grain foods are fine. But many of the foods popular among health food consumers are high in fat, saturated fat, cholesterol, sugar, and salt. These include avocados, which by weight are 44 percent fat—a fifth of it saturated. Coconut is another popular health food with a lot of fat, and coconut oil has been shown to increase the blood cholesterol level significantly. Many health food consumers champion drinking raw milk, claiming that pasteurization destroys heat-sensitive thiamin and vitamin C. This is true, but milk is not a significant source of these vitamins, and to bypass one of the most important advances in food sanitation is to risk ingesting microorganisms that can cause brucellosis and spinal tuberculosis.

The research that questions health food, in general and in certain specifics, done by those with no vested interest in denying its value, is rather convincing. But it is not to say all health food is bad, or not worth its comparatively high cost. A health food consumer is, on the whole, not going to be any worse off than the ordinary food consumer. But if there is one aspect of health food we would warn against it is the tendency of some enthusiasts to narrow the range of their diet to almost exclusive intake of grains, beans, nuts, and vegetables. Our view is that a balanced diet encompassing all the four major food groups is the essential key to good health.

23

Making a Menu

The YMCA leadership believes there is no better diet than one that comprises a balanced assortment of foods from the four major food groups. Balance is everything in making a menu, but this middle-of-the-road position need not be dull. The basic food supply is exceptionally varied, much more so than seems to have been thought when standard American fare revolved around red meat and potatoes, a boiled vegetable, a tossed salad, a hunk of pie, and a glass of milk or soda pop or a cup of coffee.

There is perhaps no better barometer of the average person's taste in food than the "fast food" restaurants, and it is interesting to note that in the past couple of years they no longer advertise exclusively the hamburger, french fries, and carbonated drink upon which their business flourished so mightily. Now featured are chicken, fish, salad bars, and certain ethnic foods.

There has been a veritable explosion of interest in trying the world's many different foods and cuisines, and not only when eating out. A mail/phone-order distributor using only television advertising sold over one million Chinese bamboo steamers in the first year after introducing the item, and maintained that sales level for the next two years. "Soul" food is no longer only for blacks, tacos are not only for Mexicans, sushi is not only for Japanese, and in many cases this expansion of the tasting experience has improved basic nutrition.

236

The four major food groups are: (1) Milk Products, (2) Beans, Grains, and Nuts, (3) Fruits and Vegetables, (4) Meat Products, which include poultry, fish, and eggs. A certain number of servings from each group every day will supply you with all the nutrients and calories you need to be healthy and active. The formula is not absolutely foolproof, though. Not all the foods in each group have the exact same amounts and kinds of nutrients. Each group is categorized on the basis of its primary nutritive constituent (meat is protein-rich, grains are carbohydrate-rich, and so on), but there is considerable overlap. Vegetables are a good source of protein, for example. Therefore, it is important to vary your food choices from each group, keeping in mind the kinds of vitamins and minerals, the amount of protein, and of course the number of calories you are taking during a meal. Charts and tables in this book will help guide you in making a menu. No one expects to plan every meal with a list of nutrient values at hand, but by going over the material periodically you will get to know whether or not you are designing a balanced menu for yourself.

What Is a "Serving"?

Before going any further you should know what is meant by a "serving," the basic measure of food portions used by nutritionists and food packagers.

In an effort to regulate the labeling of commercially prepared foods, the Food and Drug Administration ruled that nutritive values on labels had to be shown for a serving that is "average, usual or reasonable" size. That determination is left to the food packager, but the FDA has reserved the right to veto unusual or unreasonable determinations. Other FDA guidelines on the matter are that a serving must be suitable for an adult who engages in light physical activity, and that it must be shown in conventional household measures—a teaspoon, a slice, a cup, an ounce, etc.

However, because even those household measures are often vague when it comes to various foods, we want to present here some specific "serving" sizes for commonly used foods so you have something clearer to relate to when making your menu. We also include the calorie count for the items, but that does not include the number of calories you might add in preparing the food with the use of oils or fats or when adding sauces and the like to it.

A "Serving" in the Meat Group

Food	Calories
1 sm. chicken leg or thigh	90 (no skin, bone, fat)
1/2 sm. chicken breast	155
2 slices chicken or turkey, 4" × 21/4"	160
2 slices veal	120
2 slices ham	160
1 hamburger patty, 3" × 1/2"	245
2 eggs	160
4 fish sticks	160
12–18 med. shrimp	200
6 sardines	115

A "Serving" in the Beans, Grains and Nuts Group

1 slice bread	65
1/2–3/4 cup cooked cereal	60–100
1 roll, biscuit, or muffin	90–120
1/2–3/4 cup cooked macaroni, spaghetti	100–150
1 cup cooked beans, rice, lentils	200

A "Serving" in the Fruits and Vegetables Groups

1 cup raw salad, without dressing	20 or less
1 med. cantaloupe	30
10–12 grapes or cherries	40
1/2 med. banana or grapefruit	40
1 med. apple	80
1/2 cup corn	70
1/2 cup broccoli	20
1/2 cup tomatoes	20
1/2 cup beets	35
1/2 cup carrots	35
1/2 cup peas	35

A "Serving" in the Milk Group

1 cup milk	(whole, 160) (skim, 90)
1 slice Swiss cheese	105
1 cup yogurt, whole milk	150
1 cup yogurt, sweetened	250
1/2 cup cottage cheese	130

The Four Food Groups

MILK PRODUCTS (A Summary)
Daily Requirements: adults, 2 servings; children, 3–4 servings

Milk products provide an abundance of high-quality protein, all-important calcium, which is the scarcest of the minerals present in the food chain, and riboflavin, vitamin A, fat, and other nutrients. It is especially important that growing children drink milk, as their skeletal structure is forming. Adults sometimes turn away from milk, perhaps because they had so much of it as youths and feel it is a "kids' " drink, possibly because they find it too bland, or perhaps simply because it doesn't agree with them. If any of these are the case, cheese can be substituted. An adult's milk requirement can also be taken in creamed soups, sauces, custards, and ice cream ($3/4$ of a cup of ice cream is equivalent in calcium value to $1/2$ cup of milk—but the ice cream has more fat and more sugar).

For those who are watching their weight, skim milk is a perfectly good substitute for whole milk. It contains less fat, and needs to be fortified with vitamins A and D; most brands are. There are also two milk products that are a step or two above skim milk; a low-fat milk containing 1 percent milk fat, and another with 2 percent milk fat. Both are generally fortified with vitamins A and D and have a somewhat richer taste than skim milk.

BEANS, GRAINS, AND NUTS (A Summary)
Daily Requirement: 4 or more servings

This group is the prime source of carbohydrates and an excellent provider of protein that can nicely substitute for a lot of the meat we have been accustomed to eating. Americans used to get most of their protein from grains and beans and enjoyed good health. But for one reason or another meat and dairy products began to take precedence in the diet and by the 1970s were providing about 70 percent of the protein and a lot more saturated fat. Many nutritionists believe a balanced diet should derive one third of its protein from animal sources and two thirds from plants (fruits and vegetables).

Pasta, made from durum wheat refined into a white flour called semolina, has long been thought of as a fattening food and not at all the stuff of strength and high athletic performance as protein-loaded meat. Hence, before going into the arena athletes have ritually eaten a big steak. What they think they are getting is a lot of energy and stronger muscles, but protein does not produce the kind of energy they are seeking and can cause dehydration, among other things. What's more, they don't need to build up their muscles at this time because muscles do not deteriorate when used in an athletic contest. Nutritionists have begun to make these facts clear to athletes, many more of whom are now eating carbohydrate-rich pasta before the big game.

A big bowl of spaghetti provides the energy athletes need, because the complex carbohydrates are stored in the muscle tissue as glycogen. Glycogen is readily broken down into the blood sugar glucose, which is the premier fuel for muscle cells. The body has a limited capacity for storing glycogen, so it is important that an active person keep up the supply by eating carbohydrates several times daily.

Furthermore, Jane Brody has pointed out that southern Italians eat little saturated fat but lots of bread and pasta and typically have far lower levels of cholesterol than northern Europeans, who eat more red meat.

In respect to most of the foods in this group, the closer they are to their natural form when eaten, the more nutritious they are. This is especially true of the grains used in bread. The best are those made with whole grains and cereals.

When beans or nuts are substituted for other foods in this group, milk or cheese should be added to supply essential amino acids.

FRUITS AND VEGETABLES (A Summary)
Daily Requirement: 4 or more servings

Many of the foods in this group are superb suppliers of carbohydrates, but the time-honored comment of parents when putting a plate full of broccoli or spinach on the dinner table is to tell everyone to "eat their vitamins." However, if this is greeted with baleful glares (especially if the vegetables are overcooked), the family cook can get back into everyone's good graces by serving up fresh strawberries for dessert. Now everyone is happy *and* getting *more* valuable vitamins.

From this food group comes about 60 percent of our vitamin A and close to 90 percent of our vitamin C. Yellow vegetables and especially leafy dark green ones are rich in vitamin A. Yellow fruits such as peaches and apricots can take the place of the yellow vegetables. Potatoes, sweet potatoes, tomatoes, brussels' sprouts, broccoli, and all citrus fruits are *the* vitamin C providers.

Into the bargain, of course, comes riboflavin, thiamin, iron, folic acid, a good supply of water, and the all-important fiber that aids the workings of the intestines.

As we have mentioned, the "New Wave" eater has learned to steam or parboil most of the vegetables he eats in order to get superior natural taste and far more of the nutrient value. What's more, the old habit of swimming these vegetables in a pool of butter or margarine, no matter how long they've been cooked, is lessening. A sprinkle of wine vinegar or some fresh-squeezed lemon juice can enhance the flavor of these foods without fattening or oversalting them.

Eating many of these vegetables raw—celery, cauliflower, broccoli, carrots—has become a standard party "nibble" and between-meals snack; they are pleasingly crunchy and low on calories.

THE MEAT GROUP (A Summary)
Daily Requirement: 2 servings

Some nutritionists include legumes in this category—nuts, grains, beans—because of their high protein content, but most people don't think of such items as a meat dish, and besides, the protein in legumes is not quite the same.

Protein is made up of amino acids, some of which are *complete,* others of which are not. Your body needs eight complete proteins it cannot make itself, which must be gotten from meat products or from special combinations of grains and legumes, for they are not available in legumes alone. Traditionally the Western world has gotten its complete protein from cattle—"red" meat in the form of steaks, hamburgers, roasts, prime rib, etc. But we seem to be seeing a shift in this regard. Red-meat producers and purveyors are noticing a definite decline in the consumption of their products. Apparently, the considerable public discussion of red meat and its high levels of fat, along with the consequent problems of cholesterol, heart trouble, and overweight, has had an impact on the population. It is not surprising when one considers that a one-pound steak may contain 4–5 ounces of fat, 1,440 calories—a major portion of the daily requirement for the average-sized adult—and 320 mgs of cholesterol. It is ironic that the higher the grade of beef, and the costlier it is, the more fat it has.

We must have those complete proteins, 'and the newer and better sources for them have become chicken, turkey, and fish, which have much less saturated fat. However, the chicken and turkey must be eaten without their skin to have this value. Shellfish are sometimes put in the category that includes perch, haddock, and sea bass, but that is not quite correct. Lobster, clams, and oysters tend to be high in cholesterol, and organ meats such as liver and kidneys are higher still.

Red meats can be very tasty and otherwise satisfying. They need not be entirely excluded from your diet. But the best way to have your red meat, and eat it, is to go in for smaller portions at wider intervals, and/or find recipes that include small amounts in combination with other food group items.

An excellent guide to use for making up your menu has been developed by the Center for Science in the Public Interest. CSPI has broken down within each food group those items it feels can be eaten *anytime, in moderation,* and *now and then.* This scheme places the emphasis on foods generally lower in fat, cholesterol, salt, and added sugars. The foods recommended most highly tend to be richer in fiber, natural vitamins, minerals, and starches. The CSPI program is presented in Appendix 9; it can also be had as a colorful wall chart that makes for a nice decoration as well as reference. Write CSPI, 1755 S Street, N.W., Washington, D.C. 20009.

Eat for Show

Of all the living species on earth it seems man is the only one having trouble regulating his diet. Perhaps that should be narrowed down to those of us fortunate enough to have an abundance of food to choose from. Too many of us have been eating too much of what we need to live a healthy life, and eating a lot of things we don't really need which can, in fact, harm us. But we are lucky in another way, too. We have our vanity, and a poor diet shows. There may be better reasons for improving our diet than to simply make a good appearance in society, but if "good looks" is what motivates us to trim our figures with a better diet, so be it.

However, many of us who seek to improve our physical state get anxious. We take years to get out of condition, then want to make up for the neglect overnight. And there are always those among us who will try to take advantage of our urge for instant change with "miracle" solutions.

THE FALLACY OF "SPOT" REDUCING AND THE "CRASH" DIETS

There are specialists among the diet "miracle workers" who will suggest ways to lose fat in certain areas of the body, claiming that you can slim down your thighs, waist, or buttocks only and leave the rest of you as you like it. No such thing is possible. Fat cells cover your entire body. Some people have tendencies to develop high densities of fat storage cells in different body areas. When energy is needed, fat will be withdrawn from these areas, but so will it be from the rest of your body, and in just about equal proportions. That's the way the system works.

A striking illustration of the fallacy of "spot" reducing has been pointed out by Dr. Grant Gwinup, in his book *Energetics: Your Key to Weight Control*. Studies were made of the playing and nonplaying arms of tennis players which showed that while the playing arm is better developed and more muscular, the thickness of the fat layer was the same on both arms. The point, of course, is that if exercise of a particular part of the body results in the reduction of fat in it, the playing arm would be considerably less fat than the nonplaying arm. Furthermore, vibrating machines, massage whirlpools, saunas, steambaths, belts, and plastic pants may make you feel good, but they don't actually burn calories and have no real effect on reducing fat.

"Spot" reducing may not be especially dangerous, but "crash" diets promising "quick weight loss" certainly can be. These diets are inevitably based on a single "magic" food or nutrient, either the elimination of it or eating a preponderance of it. We know them as high-protein/low-carbohydrate diets, water diets, rice diets, macrobiotic diets, and countless others. Any of them are poor, if only because they mean you will not eat a balanced array of foods. You are going to miss necessary amino acids, minerals, vitamins, enzymes. These diets may have a *short-term* weight-loss effect, but over the long haul your health is threatened.

Loyola University nutritionist Elizabeth Spannhake analyzed a number of "fad" weight-loss diets. Among her discoveries was one low-carbohydrate diet seriously deficient in calcium, vitamins A and C, thiamin, riboflavin, and niacin because it leaves out bread and most milk products. What's more, the diet is overloaded with saturated animal fat and cholesterol because a low-carbohydrate diet is by definition one high in protein, and the foods people usually eat to get protein tend to be bacon, eggs, fatty cheeses, and beef.

A popular "water diet" is made up almost entirely of eggs, cheese, meat, and sugarless water. There are no fruits, vegetables, or grains.

Not only is there a severe nutritional imbalance but the diet provides no fiber and therefore is the stuff of constipation.

The awful irony of all this is that any weight loss from these diets never lasts very long, and the dieter can end up weighing more than when he or she began. This reaction has been well described by Dr. Martin Katahn, director of Vanderbilt University's Weight Management Program and author of *The 200 Calorie Solution*. Katahn has worked extensively with YMCAs in the Southeast. He works out periodically at the Y and has helped many of his clients discover the YMCA to burn off calories. Here is a much abbreviated version of what Katahn has found happens when someone goes on any low-calorie weight-loss diet *without changing his/her level of physical activity.*

First there is an immediate, large loss of body water, but very little fat. Your body begins to burn protein, and you lose muscle mass.

Your body responds to the caloric restriction and sets up defenses. Fat cells change biochemically in an effort to maintain their size and retain fat, and fewer hormones and enzymes are produced. As a result, the body's metabolism rate slows down anywhere from 10 to 45 percent. This means you begin to lose from 10 to 45 percent fewer calories while keeping your vital functions going. Your body learns to work on less fuel, and after a couple of weeks weight loss slows considerably.

At about this time people tend to start backing off their diet to some extent. This is prompted by a number of diet-related events. They feel a loss of energy because glycogen stores in the liver are depleted and muscles are not being restored, especially if the diet is one of low carbohydrate intake. You feel tired more often and have less endurance for even moderate activity, like climbing a flight of stairs. You may experience headaches and irritability because of the disruption of your bodily functions. For whatever reason, you begin to eat a bit more food. But your metabolic rate has slowed and it is now easier for you to gain weight on fewer calories than it took to maintain your vital functions before the diet program.

Whereas it may have taken 2,000 calories to maintain your prediet weight, now you can start gaining it back with only 1,300 or 1,400, *because your body has cut its needs down to the 1,200* you ate on the crash diet. As you regain weight, your body tries to readjust to your previous caloric needs—2,000. But it may not make it all the way back, and you will probably gain at least several extra pounds over your prediet weight.

Finally, because your body did everything it could to maintain fat storage while dieting, it increased its ability to conserve fat. Now it becomes highly likely that the greater percentage of the weight you have regained will be fat. If you weighed 200 pounds before you dieted and had 40 percent body fat, you may soon hit 210 pounds and have 45 percent body fat.

In brief, Dr. Katahn concludes, "never go on a diet to lose weight."

Obesity rarely stems from pathological or genetic disturbances. The simple fact is, people put on weight when they consume more calories than they use. Each of us needs a certain number of calories daily to be healthy, so the only sound solution to overweight is to be more active. However, the diet *and* the exercise do not have to be extreme. All you need is some patience, and not all that much when you consider the following.

A pound of body fat represents 3,500 calories. To lose that pound, you must burn 3,500 more calories than you consume. Let's say you eat only your daily requirement of calories, 2,500—a nutritionally balanced diet of foods from the four major groups. If you burn 3,500 calories, you lose 1,000 calories that day. At that rate, in seven days you will lose two pounds.

Statistics indicate that the typical adult male American is between twenty and thirty pounds overweight, the typical adult female fifteen to

Calorie-Burn Table

The following table lists the approximate number of calories expended per minute doing various activities, based on the participant's weight.

| Activity | Weight (pounds) | | | | |
	130	150	170	190	210
Housecleaning	3.7	4.2	4.8	5.1	5.9
Cooking	2.7	3.1	3.5	3.9	4.3
Eating	1.4	1.6	1.8	2.0	2.2
Mowing grass (Pushing gas-powered mower)	6.6	7.6	8.6	9.6	10.6
Sewing	1.3	1.5	1.7	1.9	2.1
Shopping	3.7	4.2	4.8	5.3	5.9
Sitting quietly	1.2	1.4	1.6	1.8	2.0
Card playing	1.5	1.7	1.9	2.2	2.4
Fishing	3.7	4.2	4.8	5.3	5.9
Piano playing	2.4	2.7	3.1	3.4	3.8
Painting (art)	2.0	2.3	2.6	2.9	3.2

thirty pounds over. Taking the higher amounts, on the schedule we have described you can get down to ideal weight in about four months. That is not a very long time, and you haven't starved yourself or eaten an unusual "formula" diet. Nor have you strained your body with an amount of activity far in excess of what you were accustomed to.

Remember, you burn calories even while you sleep. So to lose the thirty or so pounds over a four-month period you need only add to your normal daily activities a three-mile walk, the distance covered in around forty-five minutes. See the following table on calorie expenditure for an assortment of ordinary activities and how they impact the issue of calorie burn.

Alter Your Eating Pattern

You have made what are really rather minor adjustments to your life-style—a little more exercise, a little less food. But it is not as easy as we make it sound. If you have been doing basic things one way for a long time, changes cause discomfort. You can deflect the "pangs" of change by concentrating on the details of your altered life-style. Eating patterns are probably the most ingrained in us. To change them has at least as much to do with behavior modification as with the diet itself, because you are going to eat just about everything you've always eaten—with a few exceptions—only in smaller amounts.

You change your eating habits as much as your food. A logical place to start is with breakfast. This has probably been the "quickie" meal of your day—a slice of toast, a cup of coffee, a glass of orange juice, and off you go. The modification here is an important one. There is a saying, "Eat breakfast like a king, lunch like a prince, and dinner like a pauper." That is, you should eat a substantial first meal of the day because you have a full schedule of work (or play) ahead of you, and you need energy. At lunchtime you still have work to do and might use a bit more energy input. But it is also a time to relax, take a break from the pressure, or entertain a client or friend. You eat well. Dinner is the smallest meal since you have slowed down and will soon be asleep, but that doesn't mean it can't be a social occasion with the family. Dinner is not a pauper's meal in terms of quality, only quantity.

You might try that pattern. It will mean getting up earlier to prepare and eat a larger breakfast, but you may find the lean and hungry feeling that the light dinner has left will get you off to a spirited start.

The ideas that follow have been used successfully in YMCA classes:

• Keep a record of what you eat and drink over a one- or two-week period. Note what and how much you ate, where and when, and with whom. Figure out the calories during the daily review. The very act of recording will give your days a certain focus, a certain perspective that may reach beyond the value of diet alone.

• Eat only when you are really hungry. That doesn't mean you can't snack. And the snacks can be "fun" food. Popcorn is a big favorite with most people. Have some, but without butter, and preferably air-popped (no oil). You'll be surprised at how good it can be with only a little salt added. Popcorn is not very fattening, and it also happens to be a good source of fiber.

• Eat more slowly. Chew more thoroughly, and do not fill up the fork before the previous forkful has been swallowed. Put down your utensils periodically during the meal to talk, reflect, relax. This makes the meal more social, or sociable. Eating slowly can forestall a second serving. You will have savored the first serving, and satisfying your taste buds goes a long way toward satisfying your stomach. When you are finished eating, remove your plate or set it aside.

• Make a point of eating only in one place at home—the kitchen or the dining room. You will find yourself less prone to snacking while watching television in the den or reading in bed.

These are but a few ways you can deflect the urge to eat, modify your diet, and maintain proper weight.

Is there a diet we recommend? It should be clear by now that we advise avoiding or significantly reducing your intake of certain foods if you want to be healthier and slimmer. Basically this means cutting back on salt, sugar, and saturated fat. Eat a balanced diet of foods from the four major groups and you have a sound diet. Add to that a little more exercise daily and you have the basics needed for a fitter body.

Emotional and Mental Health

24

Exercise
for Stress Management

In 1981 the YMCA teamed up with IBM to develop the largest nationwide, multi-site corporate fitness program to date. In the first year alone over 40,000 IBM employees in 250 locations participated in fitness and stress management classes.

In 1983 and 1984 IBM loaned its corporate fitness executive, Cole Mandelblit, to the YMCA to share its experience with other companies. He spoke to top corporate leadership in seventy urban areas. The need for helping working America get in shape in order to be more productive is being felt in every type of business and industry.

The YMCA is no newcomer to this field. The organization was created in the 1850s as a response to the needs of young men who were coming to the growing cities to work in the new businesses and factories. The Industrial Revolution was creating a new type of stress. The YMCA formed groups to support each other as life-style choices were being made. But that was a century ago. We identify today with the current forms of stress—with the pressures we feel individually and collectively.

Researchers have suggested that as much as 80 percent of the common diseases suffered by the North American population is attributable to emotional stress. The figure may be a little high, but there is no denying that many millions of dollars are spent annually on tranquilizer pills meant to relieve or avoid stress, or that millions more are lost in industry through stress-related absenteeism, alcoholism, low productivity, and poor work. It is not an overstatement to say that stress is a major health and economic issue in our modern world.

A certain amount of psychological stress, in the broadest sense of the word, is a good thing, the "spice of life," in the words of Dr. Hans Selye, the so-called father of stress research. If we don't feel a degree of tension as we come close to sitting down for an important business meeting, when we make a potentially risky personal decision, or even when we tee up a golf ball on the first hole of the club championship, then we are probably not really involved in what we are doing. As a result, we may very well fail. Never to feel stress is to be without a zest for life. Stress can be a sign of creative and purposeful living.

But at what point does stress become nonproductive and harmful? Recent studies have shown that some people may be addicted to stress in the same way others are to cafeine, nicotine, or alcohol. Dr. David McClelland, a professor of psychiatry at Harvard University, has noted that "some people get a little rush of adrenalin" from risk-taking, pushing hard to win, having power over other people, "which is why they may be addicted." Dr. McClelland is describing what is referred to as the Type A personality, in which behavior is pervaded by a constant struggle against circumstances, other people, oneself, someone who approaches everything in life as a do-or-die competition. Dr. Paul Rosch, president of the American Institute of Stress, concurs that the Type A individual may unconsciously seek ways to get surges of his adrenalin coursing through his system and that he derives at least momentary pleasure from it. If the Type A personality is deprived of those surges of adrenalin, he responds like a typical addict and becomes "irritable and depressed."

The research on stress is still in its infancy. We do know, though, that it is a natural response to various life events, a fact of life from which there is no escape. There are deadlines to be met, bills to be paid, school pressures, sick children, job pressure, life changes. All these things cause stress. And while all stress is not bad and can put you on your toes and supply the energy to meet challenges, for the most part it is a negative issue, a problem when we fail to cope adequately with it. The harm is not caused by the stressful situation itself, but by our reaction to it. As Dr. Rosch concludes, "Americans increasingly seem to be living in the fast lane. A better understanding of the harm that stress can cause, as well as the possibility of some benefits, would help an increasing number of people."

We are all familiar with general signs of stress—anxiety, tension, irritability, depression—or at least the language expressing them, but there are signs of a more specific nature that are perhaps insidiously subtle. They may be actions in everyday life we may not associate with stress, if only because we are too stressed to notice them. In *Type A Behavior and Your Heart,* Drs. Meyer Friedman and Ray H. Rosenman have described a few such signs:

Moving, eating, walking rapidly
Hurrying the ends of sentences
Impatience
Guilt feelings about relaxing
Thinking about work while on vacation
Doing several things at once, such as shaving and driving your car
Trying to cram more work into ever-shorter time spans
Not listening to the opinions of others
Relating success to time—speed is everything!

We might add indigestion, a short temper over minor mishaps, and weight fluctuations to the list.

Just what the sources of stress are is being debated at length by scientists, and not many firm answers have yet evolved. It seems certain that stress evolves for some of us out of deeply rooted, uniquely personal experiences that only professional analysis can uncover. There is another source, though, that can be discerned on a relatively superficial level and is generally agreed upon. It has to do with change, especially unwanted change or change for the worse in a person's life. Change can take many forms. A well-known study of the stressful effects of change was conducted by Drs. Thomas Holmes and Richard Rahe, psychiatrists at the University of Washington Medical School.

Holmes and Rahe developed a Social Readjustment Rating Scale based on interviews with 394 individuals, each of whom assigned a mean value to a wide variety of life events after being told that getting married was equivalent to 50 points. Thus, the mean value reflects the relative stressfulness of each life event. The Holmes/Rahe Social Readjustment Rating Scale is presented below. Test yourself on it, keeping in mind that it is only a probability rating subject to any number of personal variations. Check those items that apply to you if you have experienced them in the past year or so, and total your score. The higher the score, the greater *probability* you will be subject to a health change for the worse.

The Holmes/Rahe Social Readjustment Rating Scale

Life Event	Mean Value
Death of spouse	100
Divorce	73
Marital separation	65
Jail term	63
Death of close family member	63
Personal injury or illness	53
Marriage	50
Fired at work	47
Marital reconciliation	45
Retirement	45
Change in health of family member	44
Pregnancy	40
Sex difficulties	39
Gain of new family member	39
Business readjustment	39
Change in financial state	38
Death of close friend	37
Change to different line of work	36
Change in number of arguments with spouse	35
Mortgage over $10,000	31
Foreclosure of mortgage or loan	30
Change in responsibilities at work	29
Son or daughter leaving home	29
Trouble with in-laws	29
Outstanding personal achievement	28
Wife begins or stops work	26
Begin or end school	26
Change in living conditions	25
Revision of personal habits	24
Trouble with boss	23
Change in work hours or conditions	20
Change in residence	20
Change in schools	20
Change in recreation	19
Change in church activities	19
Change in social activities	18
Mortgage or loan less than $10,000	17
Change in sleeping habits	16
Change in number of family get-togethers	15
Change in eating habits	15
Vacation	13
Christmas	12
Minor violations of the law	11

Emotional stress can make you physically ill. Some familiar manifestations include insomnia, backache, headache, asthma, ulcers, hypertension. Furthermore, Holmes and Rahe found that ten times more widows and widowers die during the first year after the death of their spouses than all other persons in their age group. And, in the year following the divorce, the divorced persons have an illness rate twelve times higher than married persons.

Clearly, illnesses resulting from stress are very real, and inasmuch as they are induced by mental or emotional forces, they can be considered psychosomatic; that is, bodily changes produced by a mental attitude. The less familiar opposite is what Dr. Selye calls somatophysics, or "the effect of bodily changes and actions upon mentality." Selye cites as an example the military insistence on the spotless appearance of soldiers as a means to strengthen morale and self-esteem. The reverse is physical degradation to break down the mental resistance of prisoners of war. Selye also recounts a personal experience to illustrate somatophysics. When he was a young boy, his grandmother, upon finding him crying one day, said, "Anytime you feel that bad just try to smile with your face and you'll see that soon your whole being will be smiling." It worked for young Selye, and later, as a doctor, he understood how a physical act can reverse a mental attitude.

There is yet another kind of physically induced emotional stress that may be the most prevalent. There is little question that when a hitherto healthy person contracts a catastrophic ailment, a bone disease, a paralysis, or something else that is clearly a physiological event, great mental stress is going to follow. But there might be less obvious changes in the body chemistry that alter metabolism or in some other way create an abnormal internal functioning and cause emotional stress. With all the research going on now in biochemistry, we should be hearing much more on this aspect of stress in the future.

We may also be victims of stress due to faulty perception or incomplete information. Perhaps you perceived from the office manager's voice that he expected you to be exactly on time for an appointment. For some reason, though, you are late and become stressed. In fact, the boss didn't mind you being late because he knew he would be involved in a troublesome confrontation during the appointment before yours. In his anxiety over that upcoming event, he left an impression he didn't really mean, and you end up paying the price with a headache, nervous indigestion—in a word, stress.

Fight or Flight

Whatever the cause of stress may be, we must learn to deal with it. In some cases the causes will suggest the cure. In other instances personalized treatment is necessary. Another means to combat stress that has wider, more generalized application is physical activity or exercise.

Exactly what happens physiologically when we are stressed? The essential response is popularly known as the Fight or Flight Syndrome, which has its genesis in earliest man. Suppose you are living in the wild, a hunter with a club as your only tool. Your only means of transportation is your legs, which, along with your arms, also constitute your primary defensive and offensive mechanisms. One day you are walking alone in the jungle and all of a sudden are confronted by a fierce, angry lion. Your whole body is immediately alerted and begins an instinctual, involuntary reaction. Your heart begins to pound, your breathing becomes shallower, and there is a significant flow of blood from your extremities into your larger muscles and the brain. The latter event is especially pertinent to Fight or Flight. If you decide to fight the lion, your large muscles are strengthened by the increased blood supply, and if you decide to run for it, the muscles will be prepared to give you utmost speed. Whether you fight or take flight, you are physiologically prepared to do the best you can. This redistribution process, by the way, is why your hands and feet become cooler under stress, and why you feel a pang or hollowness in your stomach, because nourishment is also transferred to the musculature.

In strictly medical terms the Fight or Flight Response begins in the hypothalamus, a gland in the midbrain that controls such feelings as anger, joy, sadness, disappointment, and fear. When the brain registers a danger response, the hypothalmus sends electrochemical signals to the pituitary gland located in the base of the skull. The pituitary gland secretes a hormone called ACTH (adrenocorticotropic hormone) that activates the adrenal glands. Now comes the "little surge" of adrenalin mentioned earlier. It is the release of adrenalin that brings about the physiologic changes we have mentioned—increased blood pressure, redistribution of blood, etc.

Modern man no longer needs the primitive Fight or Flight Response because he has far more sophisticated devices and methods for defending himself than his arms and legs. But his body doesn't know this yet! It is still rooted in its prehistoric past. Therefore, when a stressful situation arises, such as the threat of being fired, the breakup of a relationship, the pressure to perform well—anything perceived as being dangerous—it still elicits the rapid, rather violent changes in metabolic rate and other vital functions. It follows, of course, that the more often this change takes place, the greater the risk of developing hypertension, heart disease, stroke, and other physical illnesses.

Unstressing

The YMCA has known from experience what researchers have recently confirmed—that exercise is a powerful tool in managing stress. A California doctor once tested muscle action electrically and showed that an exercise session relaxed the muscles and slowed the pulse just as well as a dose of a potent tranquilizer. Two physiologists at Purdue University, Drs. Ismail and Trachtman, worked with middle-aged businessmen on an extensive exercise program. In the process of testing various theories about the body's responses to physical conditioning, it became increasingly clear that there were also some non-physical implications of exercise. They wrote:

"At first it was just a subliminal sense that something elusive—something that we could not measure with our stethoscopes, biochemical tests and pulmonary instruments—was happening in the course of the program. After a while we articulated what at first we only felt: we were fairly sure that our paunchy, sedentary, middle-aged businessmen were undergoing personality change, subtly but definitely. While hypochondriacal complaints were endemic at the start of the program—someone was always reporting at least one pre-heart attack symptom to us—by the time the program ended we were hearing few complaints of any type. The men often seemed to become more open and extroverted. Although many of them had known each other well before the program started, by the time they reached the end of the program they seemed to be interacting more freely and to be more relaxed. Their whole demeanor seemed to us to be more even, stable, and self-confident."

This observation led the Purdue physiologists to make specific tests of the impact of exercise on the subjects' mental/emotional condition. They first separated their subjects into one group that was already relatively fit physically and another that was not. The first analysis of test data indicated that even before the exercise program began the more fit group scored higher than the less fit group on emotional stability and imagination. After the exercise program ended, however, both groups were rated equal in these areas. The general conclusion at the end of the study was that a higher level of physical fitness was associated with such low-stress indicators as calmness and clarity of thought.

The biochemical processes that reduce stress as a result of exercise have not been definitively mapped out as yet, but some points seem clear to YMCA leaders. Regular aerobic exercises over an extended period of time result in physiological changes that help to decrease the stress response. They do so by the following mechanisms:

• Oxygen is one of the body's most important nutrients. It is required for the function of every cell. Aerobic exercise increases the body's ability to use more oxygen through developing more efficient heart and lungs and through an increased blood supply to muscles. As a result, the body develops more stamina or endurance, which allows a person to cope with stress for longer periods of time without exhaustion.

• Through increased muscle tone and better blood supply, muscles are less likely to fatigue and become sore through chronic tension.

• Changes in the nervous system help the body develop control over its alarm system. Thus, an individual's ability to cope with stress increases.

• In order to perform better, many people who get involved in aerobics become more serious about life-style modifications such as nutrition and weight control, decreased smoking and alcohol consumption. These changes also contribute to stress management.

• Aerobics, *when noncompetitive,* has been found to be useful in thought-clearing, in the release of anger, and as a natural psychotherapy for depression, anxiety attacks, schizophrenia, and anorexia nervosa *with none of the bad side effects of medication.*

In *The Work-Stress Connection* Robert Veninga and James Spradley wrote:

"We believe that exercise probably releases the tension caused by the body's mobilization for fight or flight better than any other stress safety valve. The very fact that your body mobilizes to meet stress by a vigorous muscular activity should tell you something about the value of exercise. Your blood pressure goes up to prepare you for physical exertion, your pulse rate increases to get you ready for running or fighting; your blood chemistry changes for the specific purpose of muscular activity. We interviewed a number of people who could feel the buildup of tension from their own stress response, and the healthy dissipation of that tension with exercise."

What Veninga and Spradley are saying is perhaps self-evident to many of you. Anyone who has ever gotten into prime physical condition can recall having a sense of total well-being. Such people have a strong feeling of self-control. They make decisions with less delay and with greater confidence. They feel confident that they can handle anything that comes along and that even if they are not successful because of entirely uncontrollable circumstances, they give the situation their "best shot" without undue stress both *before and after* the event. In our high-technology world a powerful physique and speed afoot are no longer the criteria that bring leadership or secure success, but good physical health still helps an individual gain the self-esteem necessary to function free of high anxiety.

The Deviation Technique

Dr. Hans Selye adds another, interesting element to the matter of stress management through exercise. He notes that mental stress is a local problem that takes place in one part of the body. Performing vigorous physical activity that stresses other parts of the body can result in a kind of tempering diffusion; the original problem is diverted.

As Selye writes, "Deviation is particularly important in combating purely mental stress. Everyone knows how much harm can be caused by worry. The textbooks of psychosomatic medicine are full of case reports describing the production of peptic ulcers, hypertension, arthritis, and many other diseases by chronic worry about moral and economic problems. *Nothing is accomplished by telling such people not to worry.* They cannot help it. Here . . . the best remedy is deviation, or general stress. By highlighting some other problem . . . by activating the whole body . . . the source of worry automatically becomes less important in proportion."

A long run, a wall-banging game of squash, a weekend of hard skiing, will divert us, make us forget a stressful emotional state. It is calming, if only because the body gets tired and wants sleep. Of course, exercise does not *solve* the problem, but it is a good way to build up a conditioned, controlled response to stress. If you become accustomed to physical stress, you will be more tolerant of mental stress. In that tolerance there is the means for becoming an all-around healthier person.

Relaxation Skills

The YMCA has developed what might be called a two-tiered system of stress management through physical activity. One is by way of vigorous physical activity—jogging, running, the aerobics we have already described. The second is the development of Relaxation Skills, a series of simple exercises that can be performed in a few minutes at your office desk or at home. These exercises focus on specific areas of the body where stress-induced physical tension often manifests—the head, neck, shoulders, upper and lower back, abdomen. There is also a Progressive Muscle Relaxation Sequence which is a variation on Relaxation Skills.

The Relaxation Skills exercises that follow should be done three to five times each, with the muscle contractions held for about six seconds and then released for at least twenty seconds before repeating. You might also use these exercises to cool down after more exertive aerobic activity.

You may want to read aloud the directions to each of these exercises, recording your voice on a tape cassette. Then play back the cassette to talk yourself through the exercise.

RELAXATION SKILLS FOR THE HEAD

Lift your eyebrows, pushing them toward the hairline as far as possible without looking up. Release, repeat.

Push your eyebrows together tightly (frown). Make as many wrinkles in your forehead as possible and hold the tension. Release so forehead is smooth again, repeat.

Slide the fingers of both your hands up into your hair. Then massage your skull by gently moving the scalp forward and back and from side to side. You can do this for as long as you like.

RELAXATION SKILLS FOR THE NECK

Sit on the floor with knees bent in front and elbows on your knees. Or sit at a table with your elbows on it. Place one hand on your cheek and lean your head and push against that hand. Resist the push with the hand. Repeat with the other hand on the other cheek. Do each exercise 3–5 times.

Clasp your hands behind your head, then pull your head up against your hands, which resist. You should feel tension in your neck. Do 3–5 times.

Take a relaxed sitting position. Then drop your chin to your chest. Now turn your chin to touch one shoulder, return it to your chest, and turn to touch the other shoulder. Hold your chin at each shoulder for about 6 seconds. Do 3–5 times for each chin-shoulder touch.

RELAXATION SKILLS FOR THE SHOULDERS

Pull your shoulders up to neck level and hold. Then pull shoulders up as close to your ears as you can and hold the shoulders tensely. Release shoulders to neck level, hold, then release shoulders completely and let your arms dangle. Do entire sequence 3–5 times.

RELAXATION SKILLS FOR THE UPPER BACK

Place your hands on your shoulders and squeeze your shoulder blades together. At the same time, press your elbows backward at shoulder level as far as they will go.

Then bring your elbows forward to touch each other in front of your chest. Relax and let arms hang limply at sides. Do 3–5 times.

RELAXATION SKILLS FOR THE LOWER BACK

Lie on your back with your knees bent and your feet flat on the floor. Relax your head, neck, shoulders, and arms. Then contract your abdominal muscles and press your lower back firmly to the floor. Hold this position, a "pelvic tilt," for about 6 seconds. Release. Do 3–5 times.

RELAXATION SKILLS FOR THE ABDOMEN

Inhale slowly and deeply through your nostrils by first pushing out your abdomen and then expanding your chest. Relax and exhale gently and completely through the nostrils by contracting the abdominal muscles lightly. Repeat so the inhalations last about 6 seconds and exhalations last longer as you become more relaxed.

Progressive Muscle Relaxation Sequence

This is another method of relaxation therapy involving learning how to recognize and then consciously release muscle tension in various muscle groups of the body. Once the ability to recognize and relieve muscle tightness is learned, it can be applied in any situation at any time of the day when tension develops.

You can do the entire sequence either while sitting comfortably in a chair or while lying on your back with your knees bent and your feet flat on the floor. This is also a good way to end a more vigorous exercise workout. Again, read these slowly into your cassette recorder. Then play it back and practice the directions that follow.

Rest your hands on your lap and put both feet on the floor. Close your eyes and keep them closed throughout the entire sequence.

Begin by slowly and deeply breathing in and out 3 or 4 times. Make your mind as blank as possible. Let yourself go limp. Continue to breathe deeply in a relaxed manner.

Now you are going to focus on various muscle groups by studying their muscle tension. Breathe in deeply as you tighten each muscle group, and breathe out slowly as you release the contraction and relax. Think about the difference in feeling between tension and relaxation.

THE HANDS AND WRISTS

Begin by focusing on your hands and wrists. Clench your hands into a fist and flex your wrists firmly. Hold the contraction for a few seconds, then let your hands and wrists go limp.

Now bend your arms, stiffen your elbows, and tighten your upper arm (make a muscle). Study the tension in your arms, then release it. Note the warm feeling of relaxation spreading through your arm.

THE FOREHEAD AND FACE

Concentrate now on your forehead and face. Frown and wrinkle your brow. Close your eyes tightly and wrinkle your nose and cheek muscles. Feel that facial tension, study it, then let it go; let the tension drain from your face.

Next, tighten the muscles of your jaw and neck and clench your teeth. Hold that tension. Then relax your jaw. Let the feeling of calmness that ensues spread through your head and neck.

THE SHOULDERS

Focus on your shoulders by squeezing your shoulder blades together and tensing your upper chest. Release this tension and let your shoulders hang limply. Sense the warm currents of relaxation flowing through your upper body.

THE ABDOMINALS

Tighten your abdominal muscles and squeeze your buttocks together. Hold the contraction firmly for a count of 6 to 10, then release fully. Do 5–10 times.

THE THIGHS

Now contract the thigh muscles by squeezing them from the hips to your knees. Hold the tension for a count of 6, then release. Note the feeling of release and growing sense of quiet in your body.

LOWER LEGS AND FEET

Focus now on your lower legs and feet. Press your heels into the floor and pull your toes up toward your knees. Hold the tension in your flexed ankles for a count of 6, then let it go.

Relax totally from head to toe and feel a sense of complete tranquillity. Hold it for a few moments. Now open your eyes.

Exercise-Plan

The YMCA believes that there are other ways to manage stress that serve as adjuncts to an exercise program. Since stress is for the most part a result of mental difficulties, it must be worked through with firm, clear thinking. YMCA classes, clubs, and camp programs emphasize these points:

KNOW YOURSELF

Your way of life should be consistent with your values, beliefs, and goals. Doing or saying things that don't agree with your inner code is a major source of stress. But if this does happen once in a while, don't be too hard on yourself. Learn to forgive yourself.

COMMUNICATE

Talk over your problems with someone you can trust. Bottling things up inside only makes things worse. Talking things out relieves the tensions, helps you to see things more clearly, and often helps you see what you can do about a problem. Remember to tell the person in whom you confide how much you value your relationship and appreciate being listened to.

TAKE A BREAK

Sometimes it can help to change the pace of your life, to escape from the problem with a book, a movie, or even a brief trip. This can help you regain your strength and balance and give you a new outlook. However, be prepared to come back and face the problem realistically. A break from routine is not to avoid problems, but to freshen your outlook and put you in better condition to deal with it.

ORGANIZE YOUR TIME AND ENERGY

Tension and anxiety build up when your work seems endless. When this happens, set priorities. Figure out what part of the day is your most productive and tackle the essential tasks then. Once those are done, you'll be in the swing of things and the other tasks will go much more easily. Don't waste a lot of energy or time on small problems. Most of what we worry about never comes to pass anyway.

BE REALISTIC ABOUT YOURSELF

People who expect too much from themselves are in a constant state of tension and anxiety. No one can be perfect. Decide what things you do well. These are probably things that you enjoy doing and that give you the most satisfaction. Put your energies into them.

Expect success and celebrate your successes. When you encounter things you don't do so well, give them your best effort and accept your own limitations. Focus on what you do well.

LEARN HOW TO LIVE WITH OTHERS

Do something nice for someone else, especially when you realize you are focusing constantly on your own problems. Ease up on competing and on edging out the other person. Rid yourself of rigidity and pride. Give in once in a while. In a race someone always loses. Cooperation is contagious; when you give people a break, they often return the favor. Life becomes easier all around.

Be easy with your criticism of others. Try to remember that all people have their virtues and shortcomings, their own values and right to be individuals. Find the good qualities and focus on them. Nurture your family relationships *deliberately*.

KNOW THAT HELP IS AVAILABLE

It does not show self-indulgence or weakness to get professional help for stress; it shows good sense. Go to your clergyman, doctor, school adviser, employer, or local Mental Health Association if you are concerned about severe, prolonged signs of stress. If you are referred to a qualified therapist, go.

25

Partnering in Feeling Good

Prior to running in the 1983 New York Marathon, a forty-three-year-old mother of ten talked to *New York Times* reporter Neil Amdur about her five-year involvement with running.

"I was a person looking for myself," she said. "I had devoted a lot of time to my family, and now I wanted something for myself."

After six months of running, weight lifting, and cycling, the woman won a 5-kilometer race. This prompted an even deeper commitment that meant training every day of the week. She felt that running made her much "sharper" at her job as a secretary and greatly improved her self-image.

"Having been a caretaker all your life, when you start doing something for yourself, it changes your attitude toward yourself," she said.

Her husband, however, was a nonrunner who felt she was devoting too much time to it *and to herself.* "I was," the woman agreed. "Running is a selfish thing. But I found a lot of personal satisfaction out of it."

The upshot of it all was that, while the children supported her running program, she and her husband divorced.

"I think my husband thought my running would go away, but it didn't."

Although we don't know the details of the relationship between the woman runner and her husband, we can use their episode in its broadest implications as a model illustrating not so much the positive effects of a physical training program, which at the YMCA we take for granted, but one of its potential dangers. We know that the success of any self-enhancement program can come at the cost of strained, or even broken, personal ties. It represents a change—a different daily routine, but perhaps more significantly, the alteration of a personality or attitude—and as we have seen, change is a primary cause of emotional stress.

Change may stir up and bring to the surface more fundamental problems in a relationship which previously were held in check by the busyness of day-to-day tasks and responsibilities. Change forces a greater honesty between people. If this, in turn, leads to a dissolution of a relationship, perhaps that is better for everyone—better than living with suppressed animosities and internalized unhappiness that can only make life joyless and bring real physical illness.

The breakup of a relationship is the most extreme eventuality of a life-style change. More often than not, however, change fosters a richer, more meaningful connection between people, one that grows and bears new fruit. This is not an automatic happening, of course, but is the result of hard work between partners. It must necessarily begin with dialogue.

Communication Is Everything

The group-work experts of the YMCA have long said that communication is everything. The mutual understanding that makes any relationship work is communication and an open atmosphere for discussion. If this does not already exist, it must be established. This can be a wrenching, perhaps painful experience when it involves change. The breakthrough is best achieved by those who feel good about themselves. It seems paradoxical, but the underpinning of meaningful, satisfactory partnering is individual self-esteem. As we have suggested, this sense of worth is given a large boost when one is in good physical health.

We all have days when we simply can't do anything right, and we feel awful about ourselves. Think about those days. Is it easy then to be thoughtful, accepting, loving? Or is it easier to be cross and irritable, especially to those who are closest to you? And what about the good days, when you've done just about everything as well as can be, when you have achieved all you have set out to do, have been complimented, and have the world on a string? We all know the answers to those questions. The point is, when our self-esteem is high, we are able to reach out to others, give love, relate well. When self-esteem is low, we cannot.

You need to increase your own self-esteem so that when there are the inevitable "down" times you recognize them and learn what you need to do to bring yourself back up. Your methods can be very simple: luxuriating in a warm bath, canceling a date and going to bed early with a book you've been meaning to read, or involving yourself in a more ambitious project, such as joining a community support group.

At the same time, you must seek to increase the self-esteem of others, to build on their positive characteristics. This takes a conscious effort that may mean holding your tongue at times, and paying compliments at other times. You must learn to send messages that build up self-esteem.

Out of this comes an environment of respect, and from this flows freedom of expression. The YMCA advocates a basic set of principles as "house rules" for effective "families" and "teams."

SPEAK FOR YOURSELF

It is your right to say what you honestly think and feel. But don't assume that everyone feels the same way. Helpful statements start with phrases like, "I feel," "I think," "I need," "It seems to me. . . ." Don't presume to speak for anyone else.

LISTEN TO OTHERS

Listen carefully and attentively to others. Show respect for their right to speak for themselves. You don't have to agree with people to listen to what they are saying. When people truly listen to each other, they begin to trust each other, learn from each other, and feel increasingly more comfortable sharing their thoughts forthrightly.

AVOID PUT-DOWNS

Verbal put-downs hurt people, even when they laugh or appear to be unaffected. Put-downs are contagious and often get thrown back. The game builds up steam, and the environment for positive communication is destroyed. If people think they might be put down, they hesitate to share personal feelings and ideas. Nonverbal put-downs—facial expressions, gestures, side conversations, even unconscious looks—also hurt. We must do everything we can to show respect for one another.

SEIZE THE MOMENT

Be tuned in to those moments when people are most apt to be impressed by what you have to say. It is not wise to speak of something new and important to someone who is in a state of depression or deeply enmeshed at the moment in his own affairs. What you have to say will only be irritating or have no impact at all, because the timing is wrong.

Trust Building

Creating an atmosphere in which there is open dialogue, where everyone feels free to express himself and herself fully, is to take a long step toward a trusting and sharing relationship. A few simple principles need to be applied to build the trust that makes relationships work fully.

Avoid negative put-downs of both yourself and others. Accept yourself and others for what you and they are.

A second factor important to building trust is that of *dependability*. When you say you are going to do something, do it!

A third factor is *consistency*. You will feel better about yourself and your relationships will be strengthened if you say what you believe and stick to your guns. Trust and confidence are hard to maintain if you say one thing one time and the opposite another time. This only causes confusion and stress. Waffling weakens relationships!

Finally there is the factor of *frequency*. The actions that produce a solid relationship must not be reserved only for special occasions—a birthday, an anniversary, or a holiday season. Trust is a layering process, a steady application of sharing, caring, and listening that forms a warm and substantial relationship.

What are some practical applications of these principles? How can you expand on these fundamentals? Read on.

Time Management

A central issue that arises in a relationship when a physical enhancement program is begun is how to fit the new activity into an already full schedule. How do you find or make the time to perform all the other things you must do in your life, and still work out? Even more to the point, will your workouts take up time you need to spend with your friends/spouse/children?

One solution derives out of the exercise itself. It has been shown that people who exercise vigorously on a regular basis need less sleep. What's more, the sleep they get tends to be more restful than that of someone who lives a sedentary existence. Which is to say, if your exercise program adds an hour or so to your awake time, you can use that time to do your workouts or perform certain duties while everyone else is still in bed. Remember, too, that you need no more than an hour of exercise a day to achieve a good training effect.

However, if you should expand your activity to a competitive level, the use of your waking hours becomes more critical. Competition and more hours of training go hand in hand.

Now it is vital that you make all your time count for something. It should be "quality" time. It is imperative that you know what you want to accomplish with every workout and that you stick to that aim. The same goes for the rest of your daily activities. Plan your days in advance whenever possible. Such scheduling tends to sharpen your concentration.

Time for relationships must be made, and this time must be made meaningful. However, it is not necessary always to "do something"— see a play, go out for a meal, whatever—nor should the pervading feeling be that being together is just another peg on the appointment board. The key to this time being "quality" is that you give it your full attention.

If the degree of involvement in your conditioning/competitive activity is great enough, however, realize that some compensations are going to have to be made regarding your commitment of time. Communications skills are vital in this event.

A young married man active with his local YMCA took up white-water canoeing and eventually became a national champion in the sport. The training to reach so high a level of achievement took substantial chunks of his time. He often got home late in the evening and left early the next morning. He missed numerous social occasions he would have enjoyed attending, as would his wife.

"But if I missed a workout," he recalled, "it would affect my self-esteem. I had set very high standards for myself, and if I did anything that might lower them, I felt guilty.

"My friends, and my wife at first, couldn't understand why the training took so much time, or why I felt I couldn't break off from it to go to a picnic or a party. I found out that if you aren't involved with the same kind of intensity, it is very difficult to understand it in someone who is. I tried to explain it to everyone as best I could. But most important, my wife was very tolerant during the long siege of training. It helped our relationship when I got her involved. She learned how to clock my times, she helped prepare my food, things like that. We would have had trouble, otherwise, and I'm not sure it would have been possible in any case if we had children."

ON-THE-JOB WORKOUTS

Another way to manage time while pursuing physical conditioning is to make use of the company fitness program. By working out on the job site, the problem of cutting into your time with personal relationships is practically eliminated. It is also, of course, another form of partnering, and a not insignificant one considering that employer-employee relations constitute a large segment of everyone's life and life-style.

While the corporate fitness program is not a new idea (the Phillips Petroleum Company began one in the 1920s), in the last few years there has been a major thrust in this direction. In 1974 there were 35 members of the American Association of Fitness Directors in Business and Industry, and in 1983 the membership had reached 3,000. The director of fitness programs for Pepsico, Inc., estimates that 10,000 corporations have instituted employee fitness programs; others believe the figure is far more than that. Companies are not setting up these programs simply as a convenience to their employees. They understand an hour or even a half hour away from the desk during working hours that is spent on exercise makes the rest of the day at the desk far more productive. It's a matter of give a little, get a *lot.*

Fortune magazine reported that in 1982 corporations spent $67 billion for employee medical insurance, and *Industry Week* added that 443 million workdays were lost in 1982, which cost business $37.4 billion. It is not certain how much those huge costs will be reduced by fitness programs for employees, but more and more corporations are betting they will. It would seem a good wager. The best study to date of the effect of physical fitness has been conducted by NASA, and it has found that when employees feel better, their enthusiasm for work increases and job performance improves. Fit employees were also found to sleep and eat better.

NASA found dramatic proof in the persons of the astronauts who flew in the Skylab missions of 1973–74. Upon the return of Skylab I after twenty-eight days in space, the astronauts were extremely weak and physically disoriented in the earth environment. Not only was there the strain of resisting gravity again after twenty-eight days of being "weightless," but their heart rate, blood pressure, and red cell count indicated they had suffered extreme physical deterioration in less than one month. What's more, it took the astronauts several weeks to regain their natural faculties.

The problem, of course, was that for all that time in space they were not using muscles or generating blood circulation against the pull of gravity. Just moving about on earth is a form of exercise, although that does not diminish the fact that man cannot live without regular physical activity. This was unequivocally proven when on the next Skylab missions the astronauts took time from their work in space to pump a stationary bicycle and walk a treadmill. When the Skylab III mission returned, after *eighty-four days* in space, their physical tests showed the astronauts to be in perfectly normal good health.

Corporate fitness programs work in various ways. Some companies offer to pick up all or part of the cost of exercise classes or membership in the YMCA. Others elect to build their own facilities and hire full-time fitness training experts or bring in counselors and trainers from organizations such as the YMCA. In Milwaukee alone the YMCA serves fifty-six corporate groups with fitness programs.

Ultimate Partnering

In Dorothy Curran's *Traits of a Healthy Family,* high on her list of the fifteen traits commonly found in healthy families by those who work in the field of human relations and family counseling is *a sense of shared responsibility.* This touches on what the white-water canoe champion found so valuable during his training—his wife's participation in the activity.

After communications and trust have been established, the best way to pursue a healthy life-style and maintain and expand a relationship with others is by joint participation. It is the ultimate expression of what we mean by *partnering.*

Self-enhancement, by definition, is an inner-directed activity that engenders apartness either in fact or by implication. In many cases the activities themselves are indeed lone-ly; people can jog or run, do calisthenics, or work out on an exercise machine by themselves. Even in a group setting this sort of isolation exists.

It is not absolutely necessary that a spouse/child/friend actually take up the activity in which you are participating, but such individuals can surely be made part of it by being enlisted to your cause. As Dr. Martin Katahn has noted, "Most families want to help the overweight member lose weight. They soon begin to see how much better he looks and feels, and they begin to reap benefits themselves. When you are happier with yourself, you tend to be happier in your relationships with others."

Thus, if you are on a fitness program that calls for less food, or a more balanced diet than the family is used to, the person who prepares the meals will not mind making separate dishes *so long as the reason for doing so is understood* and he/she is made to feel a contributor to a good thing. By the same token, if you are the cook, you must be prepared to make separate meals that suit the others. The inconvenience in either direction may vanish when the others adopt your eating plan, which they are more likely to do when not force-fed it. We are by nature social animals and tend to follow the lead of others if each of us feels we are making the decision to do so.

You might ask others to lend you a hand by keeping the records of your jogging or running times or the number of push-ups and rope jumps you perform. These are simple tasks which give your effort a concrete form in their eyes.

Question and answer games can be devised revolving around the numbers of calories in foods, nutrient values, or the musculature of the body (what is a hamstring and its purpose?). We all want to learn things, especially that which is not abstract but has day-to-day practicality.

A spiritual mood can be generated outside of a traditional religious structure by singing songs together or listening to relaxing music. This is one of the features of Dr. Herbert Benson's very popular "Relaxation Response." We might add that singing has a real physical value as well as a psychological one.

Contrary to what many people seem to think, sex life is not depressed by vigorous athletic activity. Indeed, sex tends to improve in direct proportion to how much better your physical and emotional condition is. Sex also happens to be a good aerobic exercise and has considerable relaxation value. And needless to say, sex promotes a sense of acceptance.

In the end, of course, the ideal form of partnering in a health program occurs when all the parties in a relationship do in fact take part in the activity. Even the essentially singular business of running can be a sharing experience, and not merely by running along the same path together. There is the talk of technique and equipment, commiseration over aches and pains, comparative descriptions of euphoria. Few things bring people together so well. It is the essence of team play as most of us seem to like it best. There is individual effort within the context of community. Two sides of human nature—the need to be recognized individually and at the same time as part of society—are fused into a healthy life-style. The YMCA urges you to choose a healthy life-style and stands ready to help you do it!

Appendices

APPENDIX 1

Fitness Potential for Popular Sports

Sport	Cardiorespiratory Endurance	Muscular Strength and Endurance	
		Upper Body	Lower Body
Basketball	Good	Fair	Good
Canoeing	Good–Fair	Good	Poor
Handball	Good	Good	Good
Karate	Fair	Good	Good
Racquetball	Good	Good	Good
Skating (ice)	Good–Fair	Poor	Good–Fair
Skating (roller)	Good–Fair	Poor	Good–Fair
Skiing (Downhill)	Fair	Good	Good
Skiing (Cross-Country)	Excellent–Good	Good	Excellent
Tennis	Good–Fair	Good–Fair	Good
Volleyball	Good–Fair	Fair	Good–Fair

Flexibility	MET* Range	Cal/Min	Cal/Hour
Fair	8–10	10–12.5	600–750
Poor	3–8	4–10	240–600
Fair	6–12	10–12.5	600–750
Excellent	6–8	7.5–10	450–600
Fair	6–10	7.5–12.5	450–750
Fair	4–8	5–10	300–600
Fair	4–8	5–10	300–600
Good	5–9	6–10	360–600
Good	6–12	7.5–15	450–900
Fair	4–8	5–10	300–600
Fair	4–8	5–10	300–600

*A MET refers to the rate of energy expended; one MET is equivalent to the energy needed at rest (approx. 1.25 calories, about ¼ liter of oxygen). An activity rated at 7 METS means it requires seven times more energy than a state of rest. Seven METS would be at the high end of moderate exercise; it is equivalent to 8.8 calories per minute, or a little more than 1.75 liters of oxygen uptake.

APPENDIX 2

The Ranking of Fourteen Sports and Exercises by Seven Medical Experts*

From a survey conducted by the President's Council on Physical Fitness and Sports.

	Jogging	Bicycling	Swimming	Skating (Ice & Roller)	Handball (& Squash)	Cross-Country Skiing	Downhill Skiing	Basketball	Tennis	Calisthenics	Walking	Golf	Softball	Bowling
PHYSICAL FITNESS														
Cardiorespiratory Endurance	21	19	21	18	19	19	16	19	16	10	13	8	6	5
Muscular Endurance	20	18	20	17	18	19	18	17	16	13	14	8	8	5
Strength	17	16	14	15	15	15	15	15	14	16	11	9	7	5
Flexibility	9	9	15	13	16	14	14	13	14	19	7	8	9	7
Balance	17	18	12	20	17	16	21	16	16	15	8	8	7	6
GENERAL WELL-BEING														
Weight Control	21	20	15	17	19	17	15	19	16	12	13	6	7	5
Muscle Definition	14	15	14	14	11	12	14	13	13	18	11	6	5	5
Digestion	13	12	13	11	13	12	9	10	12	11	11	7	8	7
Sleep	16	15	16	15	12	15	12	12	11	12	14	6	7	6
TOTAL	148	142	140	140	140	139	134	134	128	126	102	66	64	51

*Each expert rated components of activities on a 0–3 scale—0 indicating no benefit, 3 indicating maximum benefit. A cumulative rating of 21 for a component indicates maximum benefit from that activity.

Approximate Energy Costs of Various Exercises and Sports

From *Nutrition for Athletes: A Handbook for Coaches*. Reprinted by permission of the American Alliance for Health, Physical Education, Recreation and Dance, 1900 Association Drive, Reston, VA 22091.

Sport or Exercise	Total Calories Expended per Minute of Activity
Climbing	10.7–13.2
Cycling 5.5 mph	4.5
9.4 mph	7.0
13.1 mph	11.1
Dancing	3.3–7.7
Football	8.9
Golf	5.0
Gymnastics	
Balancing	2.5
Abdominal Exercises	3.0
Trunk Bending	3.5
Arms Swinging, hopping	6.5
Rowing 51 strokes per minute	4.1
87 strokes per minute	7.0
97 strokes per minute	11.2
Running	
Short-Distance	13.3–16.6
Cross-Country	10.6
Tennis	7.1
Skating (fast)	11.5
Skiing (moderate speed)	10.8–15.9
Uphill (maximum speed)	18.6
Squash	10.2
Swimming	
Breaststroke	11.0
Backstroke	11.5
Crawl (55 yds. per min.)	14.0
Wrestling	14.2

APPENDIX 4

The Vitamin Table

Vitamin A (soluble in fat)

Primary Sources—Dark green leafy vegetables; yellow fruits and vegetables; liver; butter and fortified margarine; cream, whole milk, and cheeses made from whole milk

Main Roles—Aids bone and teeth formation; helps form normal outer and inner skin (mucous membranes); enhances night and color vision

If Deficient—Poor bone and teeth development; deterioration of outer and inner skin; night blindness, blindness, drying of the eyes

If Overdosed—Drying and peeling of skin, rashes; loss of hair; bone and joint pain, fragile bones; enlarged liver and spleen; brain and nervous system injury; insomnia; menstrual irregularities; yellowing of skin (from carotene-containing foods—carrots)

Vitamin D (soluble in fat)

Primary Sources—Fortified milk; egg yolk; fish liver oils; sardines, salmon, tuna; direct exposure of skin to sunlight

Main Roles—Regulates intestinal absorption of calcium and phosphorous; takes a part in protein metabolism; aids in normal formation of bones and teeth, and maintenance of same

278

If Deficient—In children, rickets (stunted bone growth, bowed legs, malformed teeth, protruding abdomen); in adults, osteomalacia (softening of bones leading to shortening and fractures, muscle spasms and twitching—adult rickets)

If Overdosed—Calcium deposits in soft tissues and excessive calcium in blood; general weakness, weight loss, nausea, loss of appetite, diarrhea; kidney damage (stones); high blood pressure

Vitamin E (soluble in fat)

Primary Sources—Vegetable oils; margarine; wheat germ; whole-grain cereals; bread; liver; dried beans; green leafy vegetables; asparagus; vegetable shortening

Main Roles—Reduces oxidation of vitamin A, the carotenes, and polyunsaturated fatty acids; aids in formation of red blood cells, muscles, other tissues

If Deficient—Deficiency is rare and difficult to cause experimentally; perhaps anemia and destruction of red blood cells

If Overdosed—No conclusive evidence; possibly muscle damage and fatigue

Vitamin K (soluble in fat)

Primary Sources—Leafy green vegetables; cabbage; cauliflower; peas; potatoes; liver; cereals; egg yolk; synthesis by normal bacteria in the intestines, except in newborns

Main Roles—Blood clotting

If Deficient—Hemorrhaging in newborn children, prolonged blood clotting time

If Overdosed—Jaundice in newborn children; an excess in adults is not likely

These four fat-soluble vitamins are stored in the body, so toxicity can be built up.

Vitamin C—Ascorbic Acid (water soluble)

Primary Sources—Citrus fruits; tomatoes; cantaloupe and other melons; green peppers; potatoes; dark green vegetables; cauliflower

Main Roles—Aids in formation of collagen, the connective tissue of skin, tendons, and bone; aids formation of hemoglobin; helps protect other vitamins from oxidation; helps in the absorption and use of iron and possibly protein and carbohydrates; may block the formation of cancer-causing nitrosamines

If Deficient—Scurvy (bleeding gums, muscle degeneration, weakened cartilage and capillary walls, skin hemorrhages, anemia); early symptoms are appetite loss, irritability, weight loss

If Overdosed—May cause destruction of B_{12} in ingested food; kidney and bladder stones; diarrhea; urinary-tract irritation; can cause dependency, especially in infants if taken by mother during pregnancy

Vitamin B₁—Thiamine (water soluble)

Primary Sources—Whole-grain flours; cereals; wheat germ; seeds such as sunflower and sesame; peanuts and pine nuts; legumes such as soybeans; organ meats; oysters; pasta; bread; peas; lima beans; might be in intestinal microbes

Main Roles—Necessary for carbohydrate metabolism

If Deficient—Beriberi (muscular weakness, swelling of the heart, leg cramps, constipation); need increases if calorie intake increases

If Overdosed—No known effect

Vitamin B₂—Riboflavin (water soluble)

Primary Sources—Liver; milk; kidney; cheese; eggs; leafy vegetables; enriched bread; lean meat; beans and peas; mushrooms

Main Roles—Helps release energy from carbohydrates, proteins, fats; aids maintenance of mucous membranes

If Deficient—Cracks at corners of mouth; scaly skin around nose and ears; sore tongue and mouth; itching and burning eyes; sensitivity to light

If Overdosed—No known effect

Vitamin B₃—Niacin (water soluble)

Primary Sources—Liver; poultry; fish; wheat germ; whole-grain flours and cereals; nuts; seeds; rice; peas

Main Roles—Along with thiamin and riboflavin facilitates energy production in cells; part of coenzymes necessary for hydrogen transportation and for health of all cells

If Deficient—Pellagra (skin rashes, especially on parts exposed to sun); diarrhea; sore mouth and tongue; depression and mental disorientation

If Overdosed—Flushing of skin; sometimes jaundice; duodenal ulcer; abnormal liver function; elevated blood sugar; possible gout

Vitamin B₆ (water soluble)

Primary Sources—Whole-grain cereals and breads; liver; meats; fish; poultry; potatoes; beans; brown rice; avocados; spinach; bananas

Main Roles—Especially involved in metabolism of protein; essential for conversion of tryptophan to niacin; helps body use fats

If Deficient—Skin disorders around eyes, mouth; sore mouth and smooth red tongue; weight loss; dizziness; nausea; anemia; kidney stones; nervous disturbances and convulsions

If Overdosed—Might lead to dependency

Vitamin B$_{12}$ (water soluble)

Primary Sources—Only in animal foods: liver, meats, poultry, fish and shellfish; eggs; milk and milk products

Main Roles—Aids in formation of red blood cells; assists in building genetic materials; helps functioning of nervous system

If Deficient—Pernicious anemia (anemia, pale skin, new blood cells do not develop normally and there is a deterioration of the spinal cord that can become irreversible); numbness and tingling in fingers and toes that could lead to loss of balance and weakness/pain in arms and legs. *Strict vegetarians at risk.*

If Overdosed—No known effects

Folacin (folic acid) (water soluble)

Primary Sources—Liver; leafy vegetables; wheat germ; dried beans and peas; asparagus; broccoli; nuts; fresh oranges; whole-wheat-flour breads, cereals

Main Roles—Synthesis of nucleic acids vital to all cells; aids in formation of hemoglobin in red blood cells

If Deficient—Macrocytic anemia (red blood cells larger and fewer than normal); young blood cells do not mature; diarrhea

If Overdosed—No known effect

Pantothenic Acid (water soluble)

Primary Sources—Liver; eggs; wheat germ and bran; rice germ; peanuts; peas; widely distributed in most foods; also made by intestinal bacteria

Main Roles—Aids chemical reactions in body, particularly metabolism and release of energy from fat, protein, carbohydrates

If Deficient—Deficiency unlikely unless diet consists of highly processed foods and as part of deficiency of all B vitamins. Then symptoms include headache and fatigue; insomnia; abdominal stress; numb, tingling hands and feet; muscle cramps; loss of coordination and personality changes

If Overdosed—No known effects

Biotin (water soluble)

Primary Sources—Egg yolk; liver; kidneys; dark green vegetables; green beans; widely distributed in foods generally

Main Roles—Release of energy of carbohydrates; aids in formation of fatty acids

If Deficient—Scaly skin; mild depression; extreme weariness, muscular pains, highly sensitive skin; auorexia, and nausea

If Overdosed—No known effects

The Table of Minerals

Calcium

Primary Sources—Milk and milk products; sardines; canned salmon (with bones); dark green leafy vegetables; citrus fruits; beans and peas

Main Roles—Builds and maintains bones and teeth; muscle contraction (especially normal heartbeat rhythm); transmission of nerve impulses; proper blood clotting; enzyme activator

If Deficient—In children, rickets (stunted growth, retarded bone mineralization, poor bones and teeth, skeletal malformation); in adults, osteoporosis (brittle, porous bones)

If Overdosed—High levels of calcium in blood and urine, and soft tissues; extreme lethargy; possibly kidney stones

Phosphorous

Primary Sources—Organ meats; poultry; fish; eggs; dried beans and peas; milk and milk products

Main Roles—With calcium forms and strengthens bones; release of energy from carbohydrates, protein, fats; forms genetic material, cell membranes, many enzymes

If Deficient—Seldom in humans eating normal diet; weakness; bone pain; loss of bone calcium; poor growth

If Overdosed—Distortion of calcium-to-phosphorous ratio

Magnesium

Primary Sources—Leafy green vegetables; nuts; soybeans; seeds; whole grains

Main Roles—Release of carbohydrate energy; helps regulate body temperature, nerve and muscle contractions; helps adjust to cold weather

If Deficient—Deficiency occurs in alcoholics, people who eat highly processed foods, people who have prolonged diarrhea, kidney disease, diabetes, people who take diuretics; weakness, tremors, dizziness; spasms and convulsions; delirium and depression

If Overdosed—Disturbed nervous system

Potassium

Primary Sources—Widely distributed in foods; especially in oranges; bananas; cantaloupe, tomatoes, dark green leafy vegetables; liver; meat; fish; poultry; milk; bran; peanut butter; coffee; tea

Main Roles—Release of energy from carbohydrates, protein, fats; with sodium regulates water balance, nerve irritability, and muscle contractions, including heart rhythm

If Deficient—Rapid heartbeat; heart failure; muscle weakness; nausea; kidney and lung failure; possible deficiency occurrence when doing hard work in heat

If Overdosed—Muscular paralysis; abnormal heart rhythms

Sulfur

Primary Sources—Meat; eggs; milk; cheese; nuts; wheat germ; dried beans and peas; clams

Main Roles—Takes part in detoxification reactions; helps create firm hair, nails, and skin proteins

If Deficient—Not known in humans; a diet adequate in proteins will meet needs

If Overdosed—Unknown

Chloride (Chlorine)

Primary Sources—Table salt

Main Roles—Regulates balance of body fluids, acids, and bases as part of the fluid outside the cells; takes part in formation of gastric juices, absorption of vitamin B_{12}; suppresses growth of microorganisms in foods

If Deficient—Vomiting, diarrhea

If Overdosed—Disturbed acid-base balance

Sodium

Primary Sources—Table salt; MSG; soy sauce; baking powder; most other foods

Main Roles—Regulates water balance, muscle contractions, nerve irritability

If Deficient—Very rare; nausea; diarrhea; abdominal/muscle cramps

If Overdosed—High blood pressure (hypertension)

Iron

Primary Sources—Liver; kidneys; red meats; eggs; leafy green vegetables; dried fruits; dried beans and peas; potatoes; blackstrap molasses; enriched and whole-grain cereals; *not in dairy products*

Main Roles—Transports and transfers oxygen in blood and tissues; part of hemoglobin in blood, myoglobin in muscles, protoplasm of cells, cell nuclei, and many enzymes in tissues

If Deficient—Anemia (red cells smaller, level of hemoglobin in them lower); faulty digestion; fatigue; shortness of breath

If Overdosed—Skin pigmentation; lowered glucose tolerance; cirrhosis of the liver

Copper

Primary Sources—In most foods, but especially organ meats, shellfish, nuts, dried beans and peas, cocoa; *not in dairy products*

Main Roles—Formation of red blood cells; formation of nerve walls and connective tissue; necessary for glucose metabolism

If Deficient—In some infants fed cow milk (not breast-fed) can cause anemia; adult deficiency is unknown

If Overdosed—In Wilson's disease, a rare metabolic defect, there is abnormal storage in liver and other tissues which can cause uremia, heart defects, hypertension, violent nausea and diarrhea, death if not treated. *Cooking acidic foods in unlined copper pots can lead to toxic accumulations.*

Zinc

Primary Sources—Lean meats; fish; poultry; liver; eggs; dried beans and peas; wheat germ and bran; whole grains; milk

Main Roles—Constituent of insulin and enzymes important to digestion, protein metabolism, and synthesis of nucleic acids

If Deficient—Retarded growth (possibly "dwarfism"); retarded sexual development in children; anemia; poor wound healing; in prenatal children, abnormal brain development

If Overdosed—Nausea, diarrhea; fever; anemia; premature birth and stillbirth; bleeding in stomach.

Iodine

Primary Sources—Iodized table salt; seafood; sea salt; *vegetables grown near the sea—persons living far inland from sea should use iodized table salt*

Main Roles—Regulates the rate at which tissues breathe oxygen

If Deficient—Tissues use less oxygen, the body slows down, and eventually so do the mental processes. This results in goiter, which is enlarged thyroid with low hormone production); if mother has severe deficiency in first three months of pregnancy or before conception, cretinism in infants (retarded growth, protruding abdomen, swollen features, thick lips, enlarged tongue)

If Overdosed—If over extended period could depress thyroid activity, also causing goiter

Fluorine

Primary Sources—Fluoridated water, natural or artificial; fish; most animal foods; foods grown in fluoridated water

Main Roles—Prevents teeth decay; may also be necessary with calcium and vitamin D to maintain strong bones and prevent bones from becoming brittle and porous in later life (osteoporosis)
If Deficient—Tooth decay in children; possible osteoporosis in adults
If Overdosed—Mottling of teeth enamel; deformed teeth and bones; a fatal poison in large doses

Chromium

Primary Sources—Meats; whole grains; corn oil; dried beans; peanuts
Main Roles—Metabolism of glucose and protein; synthesis of fatty acids and cholesterol; metabolizes insulin
If Deficient—Poor use of glucose possibly resulting in chemical diabetes and adult-onset diabetes
If Overdosed—Not known

Selenium

Primary Sources—Seafood; whole grains; meat; egg yolk; chicken; milk; garlic
Main Roles—As antioxidant, prevents breakdown of fats and other body chemicals; interacts with vitamin E
If Deficient—Not known in humans; in animals, degeneration of pancreas
If Overdosed—Not known in humans; animals suffer stiffness, lameness, loss of hair, blindness, death

Manganese

Primary Sources—Abundant in most plant and animal foods; whole grains; nuts; tea; instant coffee; cocoa powder
Main Roles—Synthesizes complex carbohydrates, fat, and cholesterol; for functioning of central nervous system; normal bone structure; development of pancreas
If Deficient—Not known in humans; in animals, sterility and abnormal fetuses, bone deformation, muscle deformities
If Overdosed—Blurred speech; involuntary laughing, spastic gait; hand tremors

Molybdenum

Primary Sources—Legumes; cereal grains; liver; kidney; some dark green vegetables
Main Roles—Part of the enzyme xanthine oxidase
If Deficient—Not known in humans; in animals, decreased weight gain, shortened life span
If Overdosed—Loss of copper; goutlike syndrome

Fiber Content of Commonly Used Foods

From Anderson, J. W., *Plant Fiber in Foods,* Lexington, KY. HCF Diabetes Research Foundation, 1981.

Vegetables

	Serving Size	Total Fiber (grams)
Peas	1/2 cup cooked	5.2
Parsnips	1/2 cup cooked	4.4
Potato	1 small	3.8
Broccoli	1/2 cup cooked	2.6
Zucchini	1/2 cup cooked	2.5
Squash, summer	1/2 cup cooked	2.3
Carrots	1/2 cup cooked	2.2
Tomatoes	1/2 cup cooked	2.0
String beans	1/2 cup cooked	1.8
Onions	1/2 cup cooked	1.7
Beets	1/2 cup cooked	1.5
Turnips	1/2 cup cooked	1.3
Asparagus	1/2 cup cooked	1.2
Eggplant	1/2 cup cooked	1.2
Cauliflower	1/2 cup cooked	0.9
Cucumber	1/2 cup raw	0.8
Lettuce	1/2 cup raw	0.5

Legumes

Kidney beans	1/2 cup cooked	4.5
White beans	1/2 cup cooked	4.2
Pinto beans	1/2 cup cooked	3.0
Lima beans	1/2 cup cooked	1.4

Fruits

	Serving Size	Total Fiber (grams)
Apple	1 small	3.9
Blackberries	1/2 cup	3.7
Pear	1 small	2.5
Strawberries	3/4 cup	2.4
Plums	2 medium	2.3
Banana	1 small	1.3
Grapefruit	1/2	1.3
Pineapple	1/2 cup	0.8

Grains

Bran (100% cereal)	1/2 cup cooked	10.0
Popcorn	3 cups	2.8
Rye bread	1 slice	2.7
Whole-grain bread	1 slice	2.7
Oats, whole	1/2 cup cooked	1.6
French bread	1 slice	1.0
Dinner roll	1	0.8
Egg noodles	1/2 cup cooked	0.8
Spaghetti	1/2 cup cooked	0.8
White bread	1 slice	0.8
White rice	1/2 cup cooked	0.5

Seasoning Food Without Salt

This material used with permission of American Heart Association, Northeast Ohio Affiliate, Inc. copyright © 1978.

Meat, Fish, Poultry

Beef—Bay leaf, dry mustard powder, green pepper, marjoram, fresh mushrooms, nutmeg, onion, pepper, sage, thyme

Chicken—Green pepper, lemon juice, marjoram, fresh mushrooms, paprika, parsley, poultry seasoning, sage, thyme

Fish—Bay leaf, curry powder, dry mustard powder, green pepper, lemon juice, marjoram, fresh mushrooms, paprika

Lamb—Curry powder, garlic, mint jelly, pineapple, rosemary

Pork—Apple, applesauce, garlic, onion, sage

Veal—Apricot, bay leaf, curry powder, ginger, marjoram, oregano

Vegetables

Asparagus—Garlic, lemon juice, onion, vinegar

Corn—Green pepper, pimiento, fresh tomato

Cucumbers—Chives, dill, garlic, vinegar

Green beans—Dill, lemon juice, marjoram, nutmeg, pimiento

Peas—Green pepper, mint, fresh mushrooms, onion, parsley

Potatoes—Green pepper, mace, onion, paprika, parsley

Rice—Chives, green pepper, onion, pimiento, saffron

Squash—Brown sugar, cinnamon, ginger, mace, nutmeg, onion

Tomatoes—Basil, marjoram, onion, oregano

Soups

Bean—Pinch of dry mustard powder

Milk chowders—Peppercorns

Pea—Bay leaf, parsley

Vegetable—Vinegar, dash of sugar

From *Cooking Without Your Salt Shaker,* by the American Heart Association (available for purchase from local chapter).

Food Additives

There are seven basic categories of chemical additives.

- **Preservatives**

  One group of preservatives is the antioxidants, which prevent fats and oils from becoming rancid and stop the action that causes certain fruits and vegetables from turning brown after being sliced and exposed to the air.

  The other group is the antimicrobials, which stop the growth of molds, bacteria, and yeasts.

- **Flavorings**

  Many flavor additives are natural substances, such as citrus oils, cinnamon, and cloves. Synthetic flavors such as monosodium glutamate (MSG) have no flavor of their own but bring out the natural flavor of foods with which they are mixed.

- **Colorings**

  Some are natural substances, such as chlorophyll, caramel, and beta carotene. More than 90 percent of the coloring used comes from synthetic substances.

  If any coloring is used, whether it is a natural or synthetic substance, it must say so on the label—"artificial coloring added."

- **Texture or Thickening Agents**

  One group are the emulsifiers, which keep oil and water mixed together.

  The other group is the stabilizers or thickening agents, which give the foods a smooth, uniform look.

- **Acid Controllers**

  An assortment of acids, alkalies, buffers, and neutralizers affect the flavor, texture, and cooking characteristics. They also give flavor to soft drinks and prevent the discoloration of canned foods.

- **Leavenings**

  These include yeast, baking powder, and baking soda, which release harmless carbon dioxide into the batter or dough for bread, cakes, and other baked goods.

- **Nutrients**
  Vitamins and minerals added to increase or "enrich" foods.
  Comments on the following additives and their ratings—Avoid, Caution, Safe—are taken from the Center for Science in the Public Interest, an independent agency based in Washington, D.C. By AVOID, CSPI believes the additive is unsafe in the amounts consumed or is poorly tested. CAUTION means the additive *may* be unsafe or is poorly tested. SAFE means the additive appears to be safe for consumption.

- **Alginate and Propylene Glycol Alginate (SAFE)**
  —Thickening agents; foam stabilizer
  —In ice cream, cheese, candy, yogurt, soft drinks, salad dressing, beer
  Alginate is derived from kelp, a seaweed, and maintains the desired texture of dairy products and other factory-made foods. Propylene glycol alginate is a chemically modified algin used to thicken acidic foods and stabilize beer foam.

- **Alpha-Tocopherol (vitamin E) (SAFE)**
  —Antioxidant; nutrient
  —In vegetable oils
  Vitamin E prevents oils from going rancid.

- **Artificial Colorings, Blue #1 and #2 (AVOID)**
  —In beverages, candy, baked goods, pet food

- **Artificial Colorings, Citrus Red #2 (AVOID)**
  —On skin of some Florida oranges
  Studies indicate additive may cause cancer. The dye does not seep through orange skin into pulp.

- **Artificial Coloring, Green #3 (AVOID)**
  —In candy, beverages

- **Artifical Coloring, Red #3 (AVOID)**
  —In cherries used for fruit cocktail, candy, baked goods
  Dye may cause cancer. The FDA has expressed concern that this iodine-containing dye may also contribute to undesirably high levels of iodine.

- **Artificial Coloring, Red #40 (AVOID)**
  —In soft drinks, candy, gelatin desserts, pastry, pet foods, sausage
  The most widely used of the colorings. It needs better testing; there is a suggestion that it causes cancer in mice.

- **Artificial Coloring, Yellow #5 (AVOID)**
  —In gelatin desserts, candy, pet foods, baked goods
  Second most widely used coloring. Some people are allergic to it.

- **Artificial Coloring, Yellow #6 (CAUTION)**
  —In beverages, sausages, baked goods, candy, gelatin
  Can cause an occasional allergic reaction.
  Artificial colorings are not listed by name on labels (except Yellow #5). They are used in foods usually low in nutritional value. Some may cause hyperactivity in children.

- **Artificial Flavorings (CAUTION)**
  —In soft drinks, candy, breakfast cereals, gelatin, desserts, and many other foods
  Hundreds of chemicals are used to imitate natural flavors. Most chemicals occur in nature, but some may cause hyperactivity in children.

- **Ascorbic Acid (vitamin C) and Erythrobic Acid (SAFE)**
  —Antioxidant, nutrient, color stabilizer
  —In oily foods, cereals, soft drinks, cured meats
  Ascorbic acid helps maintain the red color of cured meats and prevent the formation of nitrosamines, a powerful cancer-causing chemical. It serves as a nutrient in drinks and cereals. Erythrobic acid (sodium erythorbate) serves the same function as ascorbic acid but has no value as a vitamin.

- **Aspartame (CAUTION)**
  An artificial sweetener in soft drinks and other foods. Aspartame, a synthetic chemical made up of two amino acids (plus methanol), was approved in 1981. While it appears safe, questions have been raised about the effects on behavior.

- **Beta Carotene (SAFE)**
  —Coloring; nutrient
  —In margarine, shortening, nondairy whiteners, butter
  An artificial coloring and nutrient supplement, it is converted by the body to vitamin A.

- **Brominated Vegetable Oil (BVO) (AVOID)**
  —Emulsifier, clouding agent
  —In soft drinks
  BVO keeps flavor oils in suspension and gives cloudy appearance to citrus-flavored soft drinks. Residues of BVO found in body fats are cause of concern.

- **Butylated Hydroxyanisole (BHA) (AVOID)**
  —Antioxidant
  —In cereals, chewing gum, potato chips, vegetable oil
  BHA retards rancidity in fats, oils, and oil-containing foods.
  A 1982 study demonstrated that it caused cancer in rats.

- **Butylated Hydroxytoluene (BHT) (AVOID)**
  —Antioxidant
  —In cereals, chewing gum, potato chips, oils
  BHT caused cancer in some studies; prevented it in others.
  BHT causes occasional allergic reaction.

- **Caffeine**
  —A stimulant
  —A natural ingredient in coffee, tea, cocoa; an additive in soft drinks
  Caffeine may cause miscarriages or birth defects and should be avoided by pregnant women. It may also cause breast lumps. Not recommended for children, because it is a stimulant drug.

- **Calcium (or Sodium) Propionate (SAFE)**
  —Preservative
  —In baked goods
  Prevents mold growth. Sodium propionate is used in pies and cakes because calcium alters action of leavening agents.

- **Calcium (or Sodium) Stearoyl Lactylate (SAFE)**
  —Dough conditioner, whipping agent
  —In bread dough, cake fillings, artificial whipped cream, processed egg whites
  Strengthens bread dough so it can be used in bread-making machinery and leads to more uniform grain and greater volume of finished product.

- **Carrageenin (SAFE)**
  —Thickening and stabilizing agent
  —In ice cream, jelly, chocolate milk, infant formula
  It comes from a seaweed called Irish moss and stabilizes oil-water mixtures. Other sources place it on the CAUTION list.

- **Casein, Sodium Caseinate (SAFE)**
  —Thickening and whitening agent
  —In ice cream, ice milk, sherbet, coffee creamers
  Casein is the principal protein in milk.

- **Citric Acid, Sodium Citrate (SAFE)**
  —Acid, flavoring, chelating agent
  —In ice cream, sherbet, fruit drinks, candy, carbonated beverages, instant potatoes
  A widely used additive, citric acid metabolizes all living organisms. Sodium citrate is a buffer for controlling the acidity of gelatin desserts, jam, ice cream, candy, and other foods.

- **Corn Syrup (CAUTION)**
  —Sweetener, thickener
  —In candy, toppings, syrups, snack foods, imitation dairy foods
  A sweet, thick liquid made by treating cornstarch with acids or enzymes, it contains no nutritional value other than calories.

- **Dextrose (Glucose, Corn Sugar) (CAUTION)**
  —Sweetener, coloring agent
  —In bread, caramel, soda pop, cookies, many other foods
  An important chemical in every living organism, dextrose is a natural sugar that is the source of sweetness in fruits and honey. As an additive, it adds empty calories. Also, as it turns brown when heated, dextrose contributes to the color of bread crust and toast.

- **EDTA (SAFE)**
  —A chelating agent
  —In salad dressings, margarine, sandwich spreads, mayonnaise, processed fruit and vegetables, canned shellfish, soft drinks
  Modern food manufacturing involves metal rollers, blenders, and containers that result in trace amounts of metal contamination in foods. EDTA (ethylenediaminete-traacetic acid) traps metal impurities which would promote rancidity and break down artificial colorings.

- **Ferrous Gluconate (SAFE)**
  —Coloring, nutrient
  —In black olives
  Used to create a uniform jet-black color in black olives. In pill form it is a source of iron.

- **Fumaric Acid (SAFE)**
  —Tartness agent
  —In powdered drinks, pudding, pie fillings, gelatin desserts
  A source of tartness and acidity in dry food products.

- **Gelatin (SAFE)**
  —Thickening and gelling agent
  —In powdered dessert mix, yogurt, ice cream, cheese spreads, beverages
  A protein derived from animal bones, hooves, and other parts, it has little nutritional value.

- **Glycerin (Glycerol) (SAFE)**
  —Maintains water content
  —In marshmallows, candy, fudge, baked goods
  Glycerin is the backbone of fat and oil molecules. The body uses it as a source of energy or to catalyze more complex molecules into being. It is quite safe.

- **Gums (guar, locust bean, arabic, furcelleran, ghatti, karaya, tragacanth) (SAFE)**
  —Thickening agents, stabilizers
  —In beverages, ice cream, frozen puddings, salad dressing, dough, cottage cheese, candy, drink mixes
  Gums derived from natural sources (bushes, trees, seaweed) are used to thicken foods, to prevent sugar crystals from forming in candy, to stabilize beer foam, and to keep oil and water mixed in salad dressing.

- **Heptyl Paraben (CAUTION)**
  Preservative
  —In beer
  Studies suggest it is safe, but tests have not been done in the presence of alcohol.

- **Hydrogenated Vegetable Oil (CAUTION)**
  —Source of oil or fat
  —In margarine and many processed foods
  Vegetable oil is usually a liquid, but it can be made into a semisolid by treating it with hydrogen. However, hydrogenation converts some of the polyunsaturated oil to saturated fat.

- **Hydrolyzed Vegetable Protein (HVP) (SAFE)**
  —A flavor enhancer
  —In instant soups, frankfurters, sauce mixes, beef stew
  Consists of a vegetable protein (usually soybean) that has been chemically broken down.

- **Invert Sugar   (CAUTION)**
  —A sweetener
  —In candy, soft drinks, numerous other foods
  —A mix of two sugars, dextrose and fructose, it is sweeter and more soluble than sucrose (table sugar). Provides empty calories, causes tooth decay.

- **Lactic Acid   (SAFE)**
  —Acidity regulator
  —In Spanish olives, cheese, frozen desserts, carbonated drinks
  A safe acid that occurs in almost all living organisms, it inhibits spoilage in Spanish-type olives, balances acidity in cheese-making, adds tartness to frozen desserts, carbonated fruit-flavored drinks, and other foods.

- **Lactose   (SAFE)**
  —A sweetener
  —In whipped topping mix, breakfast pastry
  A carbohydrate found only in milk, it is one-sixth as sweet as table sugar. Milk turns sour when bacteria convert lactose to lactic acid. Non-Caucasians may have trouble digesting lactose.

- **Lecithin   (SAFE)**
  —Emulsifier, antioxidant
  —In baked goods, margarine, chocolate, ice cream
  A common component of animal and plant tissues, it is a source of choline. It keeps oil and water from separating, retards rancidity, reduces spattering in the frying pan, leads to fluffier cakes.

- **Mannitol   (SAFE)**
  —A sweetener, and other uses
  —Chewing gum, low-calorie foods
  Not as sweet as sucrose (it contributes about half as many calories), mannitol is used as "dust" on chewing gum. It prevents gum from absorbing moisture and becoming sticky.

- **Mono- and Diglycerides   (SAFE)**
  —Emulsifier
  —In baked goods, margarine, candy, peanut butter
  Makes bread softer and prevents staling, improves stability of margarine, makes caramels less sticky, keeps oil in peanut butter from separating out. Most foods in which mono- and diglycerides are used tend to be high in refined flour, sugar, or fat.

- **Monosodium Glutamate (MSG)   (CAUTION)**
  —Flavor enhancer
  —Soup, seafood, poultry, cheese, sauces, stews, other foods
  An amino acid that brings out the flavor of protein-rich foods, large amounts fed to infant mice destroyed nerve cells in the brains. Public pressure forced baby-food manufacturers to stop using MSG. For children it is an (AVOID). May cause headaches.

- **Phosphoric Acid; Phosphates   (CAUTION)**
  —Acidulant, chelating agent, buffer, emulsifier, nutrient, discoloration inhibitor
  —In baked goods, cheese, powdered foods, cured meat, soda pop, breakfast cereals, dehydrated potatoes
  Phosphoric acid acidifies and flavors cola drinks. Phosphate salts are used extensively in many processed foods. Calcium and iron phosphates are mineral supplements; sodium aluminum phosphate is a leavening agent; calcium and ammonium phosphates serve as bread yeast; sodium acid pyrophosphate prevents the discoloration of potatoes and sugar syrups. Phosphates are not toxic, but extensive use of them has led to dietary imbalance that may be causing osteoporosis, a bone disease suffered by adults.

- **Polysorbate 60, 65, and 80   (CAUTION)**
  —An emulsifier
  —In baked goods, frozen desserts, imitation dairy products
  They are sometimes contaminated with 1,4-dioxane, a carcinogenic. They keep baked goods from going stale, dill oil from dissolving in bottled pickles, helps coffee whiteners dissolve in coffee, prevents oil from separating out of artificial whipped cream.

- **Propyl Gallate   (AVOID)**
  —An antioxidant
  —In vegetable oil, meat products, potato sticks, chicken soup base, chewing gum
  Retards spoilage of fats and oils. It is often used with BHA and BHT because the combination retards rancidity. Recent study suggested (but did not prove) Propyl Gallate promotes cancer.

- **Quinine   (AVOID)**
  —Flavoring
  —Tonic water, quinine water, bitter lemon
  Can cure malaria and gives a bitter flavoring to a few soft drinks. Pregnant women should avoid quinine-containing drugs and drinks, as large amounts may cause birth defects.

- **Saccharin (AVOID)**
  An artificial sweetener in soft drinks and other foods. It is 350 times sweeter than sugar. Studies have not shown that it helps people lose weight. In 1977 FDA proposed that it be banned, because of repeated evidence that it causes cancer. It is gradually being replaced by Aspartame.

- **Salt (Sodium chloride) (AVOID)**
  —Flavoring
  —Most processed foods
  Diets high in salt and other sources of sodium promote high blood pressure, a major cause of heart attack and stroke.

- **Sodium Benzoate (SAFE)**
  —In fruit juice, carbonated drinks, pickles, preserves
  It has been used for over seventy years to prevent the growth of microorganisms in acidic foods.

- **Sodium Carboxymethylcellulose (SAFE)**
  —Thickening and stabilizing agent
  —In ice cream, beer, pie fillings, icings, diet foods, candy
  CMC is made by reacting cellulose with an acetic acid derivative. It also prevents sugar from crystalizing.

- **Sodium Nitrite, Sodium Nitrate (AVOID)**
  —Preservative, coloring, flavoring
  —In bacon, ham, frankfurters, luncheon meats, smoked fish, corned beef
  One of the most controversial additives, especially because it is used in so many favorite foods, sodium nitrite is coming into greater and greater disfavor because of its potential for introducing a slight risk of cancer. The U.S. Department of Agriculture has made mandatory the reduction of nitrites and nitrates in certain products, and the total elimination of nitrites in others. What's more, the department has specified that even the reduced amount of nitrite in bacon must be used with sodium ascorbate to block the formation of nitrosamines; fried bacon is particularly prone to this. Nitrosamines are cancer-causing chemicals formed when nitrites combine with food substances called amines, which are prominent in meat and fish.
  Nitrite is what gives bacon, corned beef, and hot dogs a red color. Bacon and corned beef would otherwise be brown, hot dogs a kind of gray. The additive also gives the flavor to these foods that we have become accustomed to.
  The chief value of nitrite is that it prevents botulism, a bacterial poisoning. This is obviously valuable, but antinitrite proponents feel research should be stepped up to find another botulism preventative without the carcinogenic potential of nitrite.
  Sodium nitrate is used in dry-cured meat because it slowly breaks down into nitrite.

- **Sorbic Acid, Potassium Sorbate (SAFE)**
  —Prevents growth of mold and bacteria
  —In cheese, syrup, jelly, cake, wine, dry fruits
  Sorbic acid occurs naturally in the berries of the mountain ash.

- **Sorbitan Monostearate   (SAFE)**
  —An emulsifier
  —In cakes, candy, frozen pudding, icing
  The additive keeps oil and water mixed together. In chocolate candy it prevents discoloration that occurs when candy is warmed then cooled.

- **Sorbitol   (SAFE)**
  —A sweetener, thickening agent, maintains moisture
  —In dietetic drinks and foods, candy, shredded coconut, chewing gum
  Sorbitol occurs naturally in fruits and berries. It is half as sweet as sugar. It is used in noncariogenic (anticavity) chewing gum because oral bacteria do not metabolize it well. Large amounts of sorbitol have a laxative effect on adults. Diabetics use it because it is absorbed slowly and does not cause blood sugar to rise rapidly.

- **Starch, Modified Starch   (SAFE)**
  —A thickening agent
  —In soup, gravy, baby foods
  Starch by itself is a thickening agent. But it does not dissolve in cold water, so chemists have mixed it with various chemicals, and in this modified form it improves the consistency of some foods and keeps solids suspended. Starch and modified starch make foods look thicker than they really are.

- **Sugar (Sucrose)   (AVOID)**
  —A sweetener.
  —Table sugar, and in many, many processed foods
  The best promoter of tooth decay may also promote obesity. We're eating too much of it.

- **Sulfur Dioxide, Sodium Bisulfite   (AVOID)**
  —A preservative and bleach
  —In sliced fruit, wine, grape juice, dehydrated potatoes
  Sulfur dioxide is a gas; sodium bisulfate is a powder. They prevent the discoloration of dried apricots, apples, and similar foods. They prevent bacterial growth in wine and other foods. "Sulfiting agents" have caused fatal reactions in asthmatics—the only current additive known to have killed people. They destroy vitamin B_1, hence the (AVOID) designation.

- **Vanillin, Ethyl Vanillin   (SAFE)**
  —A substitute for vanilla
  —In ice cream, baked goods, beverages, chocolate, candy, gelatin desserts
  True vanilla flavoring is derived from a bean. Vanillin, the major flavor component of vanilla, is cheaper to produce synthetically. Ethyl vanillin is a derivative of vanillin and comes nearer to the taste of real vanilla.

"The New American Eating Guide"

Food Group	Anytime	In Moderation	Now and Then
Beans, Grains, and Nuts	bread and rolls, whole grain bulghur dried beans and peas lentils oatmeal pasta, whole wheat rice, brown rye bread sprouts (bean, alfalfa) whole-grain hot and cold cereals whole-wheat matzoh	corn bread[8] flour tortilla[8] granola cereals[1 or 2] hominy grits[8] macaroni and cheese[1,(6),8] matzoh[8] nuts[3] pasta, regular[8] peanut butter[3] pizza[6,8] refined, unsweetened cereals[8] refried beans[1,2] seeds[3] soybeans[2] tofu (bean curd)[2] waffles/pancakes with syrup[5,(6),8] white bread and rolls[8] white rice[8]	croissant[4,8] doughnut, yeast-leavened[3 or 4,5,8] presweetened breakfast cereal sticky buns[1 or 2,5,8] stuffing, made with butter[4,(6),8]

[1]—moderate fat, saturated   [2]—moderate fat, unsaturated   [3]—high fat, unsaturated   [4]—high fat, saturated   [5]—high in added sugar   [6]—high in salt or sodium   [(6)]—may be high in salt or sodium   [7]—high in cholesterol   [8]—refined grains

Food Group	Anytime	In Moderation	Now and Then
Fruits and Vegetables	All fruits and vegetables except those listed at right applesauce, unsweetened vegetable juices, unsalted potatoes, white or sweet	avocado[3] coleslaw[3] cranberry sauce, canned[5] dried fruit french fries, homemade in vegetable oil;[2] commercial[1] fried eggplant (vegetable oil)[2] fruits canned in syrup[5] gazpacho[2,(6)] glazed carrots[5,(6)] guacamole[3] potatoes au gratin[(6)] vegetable juices, salted[6] fruit juices, sweetened[5] vegetables canned with salt[6]	coconut[4] pickles[6]
Milk Products	skim buttermilk low-fat yogurt and fruit juice drink (lassi) low-fat cottage cheese low-fat milk (1% milk fat) low-fat yogurt nonfat dry milk skim-milk cheeses skim milk skim milk and banana shake	cocoa made with skim milk[5] cottage cheese, regular, 4% milk fat[1] frozen low-fat yogurt[5] ice milk[5] low-fat milk (2% milk fat)[1] low-fat yogurt, sweetened[5] mozzarella cheese, part skim only[(6)]	cheesecake[5] cheese fondue[4,(6)] cheese soufflé[4,(6),7] eggnog[1,5,7] hard cheeses: blue, brick, Camembert, cheddar, Swiss, Muenster[4,(6)] ice cream[4,5] processed cheeses[4,6] whole milk[4] whole-milk yogurt[4]
Poultry, Fish, Meat, and Eggs	cod gefilte fish[(6)] flounder haddock halibut perch pollock rockfish shellfish, except shrimp sole	fried fish[1 or 2] herring[3,6] mackerel, canned[2,(6)] salmon, pink, canned[2,(6)] sardines[2,(6)] shrimp[7] tuna, oil-packed[2,(6)] chicken liver[7] fried chicken, homemade in	fried chicken, commercial[4] cheese omelet[4,7] egg yolk or whole egg (3 a week) bacon[4,(6)] beef liver, fried[1,7] bologna[4,6] corned beef[4,6] ground beef[4] ham, well trimmed[1,6]

Food Group	Anytime	In Moderation	Now and Then
	tuna, packed in water	vegetable oil[3]	hot dogs[4,6]
	egg whites only	chicken and turkey, boiled, baked, roasted (w/skin)[2]	liverwurst[4,6]
	chicken and turkey, boiled, baked, roasted (no skin)	flank steak[1]	pig's feet[4]
		leg/loin of lamb[1]	salami[4,6]
		pork shoulder or loin, lean[1]	sausage[4,6]
		steak, round or ground round[1]	spareribs[4]
		rump roast[1]	red meats, untrimmed[4]
		steak, sirloin, lean[1]	
		veal[1]	

[1]—moderate fat, saturated [2]—moderate fat, unsaturated [3]—high fat, unsaturated [4]—high fat, saturated [5]—high in added sugar [6]—high in salt or sodium (6)—may be high in salt or sodium [7]—high in cholesterol [8]—refined grains

Index

303